CW01265934

The Heart Club

A history of London's heart surgery pioneers

Tom Treasure

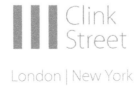

London | New York

Published by Clink Street Publishing 2017
Copyright © 2017
First edition.
The author asserts the moral right under the Copyright, Designs and Patents Act 1988 to be identified as the author of this work.
All rights reserved. No part of this publication may be reproduced, stored in a retrieval system or transmitted, in any form or by any means without the prior consent of the author, nor be otherwise circulated in any form of binding or cover other than that with which it is published and without a similar condition being imposed on the subsequent purchaser.
ISBN: 978-1-911525-84-4 paperback, 978-1-911525-85-1 ebook

*To the memory of the doctors of the
Peacock Club and their patients.*

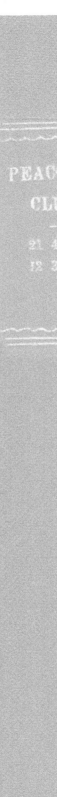

Contents

Preface	1
Peace returns to Guys Hospital 1945–1948	7
The Minutes of the Peacock Club 1948–1956	35
Three Blue Babies – their lives 1944–2017	185
Biographical Notes: List 1	217
Author networks	243
Biographical Notes: List 2	247
Glossary of terms and notes on the minutes	261
Abbreviations	277
Reference List	281
About Tom Treasure	303

Acknowledgements

Many people have helped me in conversations, as sources of information and in reflection on where the events in this book sit not only in the history of medicine but in social history and humanity. Most of the many who helped me are listed formally in the Preface. Those I might have forgotten, please feel included in my gratitude for helping me in this task which has been the product of years of deliberation. Particularly I thank John Chambers for finding the book, Christopher Lawrence for mentoring me and Caroline Coates who curates the Arthur Hollman Collection at the British Cardiovascular Society and has taken the Minutes of the Peacock Club into safe keeping

I am especially grateful to Gareth, Hayley, Josh and Kate at Clink Street for guiding this book into print.

Preface

Central to this book are the Minutes of the Peacock Club. These are the consecutive accounts of 47 meetings in Guys Hospital from April 1947 to March 1956. They are in a small bound volume which is now in the historical collection of the British Cardiovascular Society in Fitzroy Square in London. The volume was found by Dr John Chambers among books and papers on the shelves of Guys cardiology department. The building, the old Hunts House, was demolished not long afterwards and the Minutes might easily have been lost had John Chambers not saved them.

The work of the Peacock Club is recorded in the Minutes of 47 meetings from 1948 to 1956 but as to the history of the volume itself I am left guessing. The bound volume is made up of several exercise books with ruled pages. Some of the earlier minutes were hand written. Later they were more often typed and pasted onto the pages. The minutes clearly antedate the binding because in several instances, marginal content has been lost due to cropping in the binding process. The Minutes were routinely signed and dated. The date on which they were signed matches that of the next meeting, so they are consecutive. The last Minute is for March 1956 and is unsigned; it appears that there was no subsequent meeting at which to sign them. The year coincides with Maurice Campbell retiring from Guys Hospital. From then, who was the custodian of the Minutes and who had them bound? At this point I do not know.

In 1951 in the first few years of the Club Russell Brock wrote:

> Intracardiac surgery is not for the lone worker. Team work is essential. To give one example, at Guys there is a group of some 15 people actively engaged in the work, and as time passes we find that more and more are drawn into the team.[1]

1

The Heart Club

The group he refers to was the Peacock Club. But why the name Peacock? It is explained in the first few meetings. The Club was named after Dr Thomas Peacock. In his 1858 book on malformations of the human heart[2] he gave a clear description of the four components of the congenital malformation, generally known as Fallots Tetralogy.

As a guide to navigating this book the headings below indicate the contents of the successive chapters. The chapters are interrelated to some degree but are self-contained and do not have to be read consecutively.

Peace returns to Guy's Hospital 1945–1948

This first chapter sets the scene in London 1945 when Guys Hospital began to function normally again. The medical and outpatient work of the hospital returned from Orpington in Kent where it had been since 1939 under the leadership of Dr Maurice Campbell. Russell Brock had remained in London while the hospital suffered bombing and fire damage. Campbell and Brock are central to this story. From the relative safety of Tunbridge Wells, the students and preclinical teachers of the medical school came back to Guys. Dr Boland, back from the North African theatre of war, was made their Dean. He immediately set about establishing exchange visits for the clinical teachers with Johns Hopkins Hospital in Baltimore, the first of whom was Alfred Blalock. The chapter closes with the founding of the Peacock Club.

The Minutes of the Peacock Club 1948–1956

The Minutes of the 47 meetings have been transcribed and presented complete. Footnotes signpost further information and explanations in the look-up lists near the end of the book but the Minutes largely speak for themselves. The full contents of the Minutes, in their original appearance, are available as .jpg files from the archive of the British Cardiovascular Society. I have therefore made an editorial decision to present an easy to read version of what the writers of the Minutes intended to be understood, rather than struggling to attempt a facsimile through modern software. So I have not reproduced typographical errors, the forensic evidence of hand written corrections, variations in punctuation, or obvious spelling errors. But contemporary usual spelling and usages have been preserved, for example the alternative spelling of shew for our usual show has not been changed. Where there are possible uncertainties, such as the identity of individual names due to spelling variations in the original, this is indicated. There remains some variation in the format of the minutes reflecting the variety of hands that played a part in keeping the record. Selected pages are interposed as scanned images of the original and there are illustrations from contemporary publications.

The meeting headlines I have provided at the beginning of the Minutes suggest three overlapping phases of the meetings. At first, they were getting organised and learning how to select and investigate patients for operations which were new and experimental. In the middle phase, they were presenting their on-going laboratory and clinical research. In the third phase, there were studies of the outcomes of their operations. Throughout the Minutes there are presentations of clinical cases for the team to review so they could improve their selection and operations. Research work was presented in preparation for its publication. By tracing the authors and their written output we can track the stages of dissemination from *Guy's Hospital Reports*, through the *British Heart Journal* and the *British Medical Journal* to specialist and international journals.

Three 'Blue Babies'– their lives

I have been fortunate to have met and to work with three remarkable people who were treated for congenital heart disease in the 1950s – John Hunt, Xerxes Talati and Geraldine West. They tell their own life stories. I am grateful to Dr Kate Bull for introducing me to them.[3] Through their sometimes complicated lives they all were treated at some stage by doctors of the Peacock Club. Their stories chart the developments, and some of the sequelae of this earliest surgery for congenital heart disease, up to the present day.

Biographical Notes: Lists 1 and 2

The first two (of five) look-up lists are brief biographies. List 1 is of those who attended the club. As Brock wrote in 1951 there was a nucleus of about 15 people actively engaged in the work at any particular time.[1] Who these

The Heart Club

people were evolved as new members of staff were appointed and trainees, residents, clinical and research staff came and went. As a result, outside the nucleus of 15 or so, many were young, in their mid-twenties to early thirties. There were over 40 attendees as members, of which only two were women. In addition, nearly 50 visitors are named. In the later years, attendance lists were not kept so there were probably many more occasional visitors.

At the end of the list there is a graphical depiction of a network analysis illustrating the extensive research collaborations between the members and other attendees.

Biographical Notes List 2 is of people named in the minutes and whose work was cited. Many of them made large lifetime contributions so I have limited the information to matters pertaining to the Clubs discussions and provided references and sources for further reading.

Glossary of Terms and Notes on the Minutes
The third of the look-up lists is a gallimaufry, but in alphabetic order, of some things that seem to me to need some explanation. I have sometimes found in explanatory notes explanations of everything apart from the one thing you need to know but I have done my best to provide sufficient information and not too much. Medical readers will not need the explanation of standard medical terms. Specialist medical readers may be tempted to dismiss or reinterpret what was written in the Minutes but that would be to miss the point, and I urge readers to resist that temptation. I have tried to be fastidious in explaining what the Club understood by these terms in 1948–1956 so I use contemporary texts and explanations. For example, the contemporary Guys text book of medicine was the multi-author book edited by the senior physician Sir John Conybeare. Dr Maurice Campbell contributed the chapter on heart disease, so this represents what was known, believed and practised at the time of the Peacock Club.[4,5] Remember that seventy years into the future, many of our medical beliefs and practices will be seen differently then.

List of Abbreviations
This fourth look-up list spells out the abbreviations used in the Minutes and the Biographical Notes.

References
The fifth look-up list is of published writings cited in the book. The list is compiled in the way that I am familiar with in medical science. It may be irksome for historians, more used to footnotes and end notes. There are some footnotes but they are intentionally brief and any that refer to external sources lead to this single list of available published work at the end of the book.

In compiling these five look-up lists I took my lead from Raymond Hurt whose *History of Cardiothoracic Surgery* has several chronological or alphabetical lists of subjects and writers.[6] As a result, of all the books of history of medicine on my own shelves, his book is the one I look up most often. I can find what I am looking for more often than not. I hope my lists will serve that purpose.

Acknowledgements
I am grateful to many people for help in reaching a better understanding of the Peacock Club and researching its members and guests. First and foremost, my thanks go to Christopher Lawrence an academic historian who was my supervisor and mentor during my four month mid-career sabbatical in History of Medicine at the Wellcome Institute in 1994–1995. I showed him the rediscovered Minutes of the Peacock Club that long ago. Without his impetus I would not have embarked on the project of publishing them in an accessible form for all to read. To quote from the Minutes *March 1951*: Mr Brock remarked that it was easy to go on finding objections, the thing was to get on with the job. Chris Lawrences extensive knowledge of mid-twentieth-century history was invaluable particularly in his contributions made in compiling the Biographical Notes List 2.

Of the many others who have helped me, I will have forgotten some for which I apologise but these I thank individually: Torkel Åberg, Robert Anderson,

The Heart Club

Hana Barrett, Jessica Borge, Kate Bull, Raphael Caldeira, John Chambers, Kenneth Citron, Caroline Coates, the late Laurence Cohn, Jules Dussek, Ian Earl, William Edwards, Sir Terence English, Sandra Gabriel, Julie Grahame, the late Arthur Hollman, Raymond Hurt, Richard Hurvitz, Sir Barry Jackson, Marjorie Kehoe, Christopher Lincoln, the late Edward Mansell, Richard Meunier, Mark Monks, Tom Nellist, John Pepper, Michael Purton, Piers Reinhold, Barry Ross, Rosina Sharrock, Jane Somerville, Lianne Smith, Jaroslav Stark, John Stephens, the late Marvin Sturridge, Caroline Tindall and Joe Treasure. I was helped by the staff of various archives and libraries, namely: Alan Mason Chesney Archives of the Johns Hopkins Medical Institutions, British Cardiovascular Society, British Library, Cirencester Public Library, Countway Library Harvard Medical School, the Estate of Yousuf Karsh, Express Newspapers, Gordon Museum, James Lind Library, Kings College London Archives, Lillian & Clarence de la Chapelle Archives of NYU and Bellevue Hospitals, New York, London Metropolitan Archive, Royal Society of Medicine, Wellcome Library and Wilts and Gloucestershire Standard. *Munk's Roll of the Fellows of the Royal College of Physicians* and *Parr's Lives of the Fellows of the Royal College of Surgeons* have been invaluable.

Peace returns to Guy's Hospital 1945–1948

The wartime bombardment

May 12th 1945 *Guy's Hospital Gazette* published a picture of the statue of Thomas Guy, the hospitals patron, being disinterred from the concrete that had encased it for the duration of the war.[7] Dr Peter Bishop had been Medical-Officer-in-Charge of the hospital which had been run as part of the wartime Emergency Medical Service. He had been just 35 years old when the war started. There is something darkly humorous about his laconic style in the article he wrote for the *Gazette* in July 1945 detailing the air bombardment that severely affected Guys.[8] The bombing started in earnest in September 1940, about a year after war was declared.

> On September 7th the blow was struck at last. High in the clear sky of a glorious summer evening three hundred and fifty German bombers and fighters flew up the Thames and dropped their bombs on the London Docks.

Guys is immediately adjacent to the site of those docks. It was itself repeatedly bombed while at the same time receiving those injured in the vicinity. Peter Bishop describes the various phases of the bombardment including the flying bombs, the propeller driven V1 pilotless planes which were particularly terrifying.

> We had certainly expected something unpleasant to happen shortly before or shortly after D-Day, but, of course, we didnt expect flying bombs. Indeed we didnt know what they were when they first arrived; nor did we know how to cope with them, and here we were in good company, for the Governments order to shoot them down even in the heart of London brought us in over three hundred casualties in the first week.

7

GUY'S HOSPITAL GAZETTE
A Journal of Medicine, Surgery, Dentistry and Hospital News
PUBLISHED FORTNIGHTLY

Vol. LIX   No. 1482   12th May, 1945   Ninepence

PASSIM

THIS fortnight has seen the long-awaited unveiling of Thomas Guy from his tomb of concrete, the first statue to be uncovered in London. This arising is, we hope, symbolical of the rising of a new Guy's from the dust of the old; now that peace is upon us, we anticipate that the plans for rebuilding will go on apace. Thomas Guy himself, though rather dusty after his five years' incarceration, appears otherwise none the worse for it and we must praise the foresight of those who thus enclosed him. Several photographs of the disinterrment were obtained, some depicting our worthy patron in rather undignified circumstances, and we are reproducing one of these in this issue.

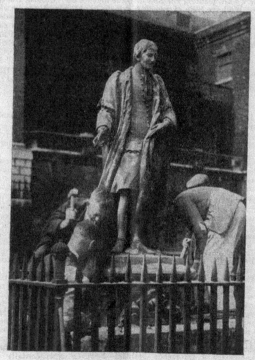

By kind permission of Fox Photos Ltd.

The statue of Thomas Guy had spent the war encased in concrete. On 12th May 1945 Guys Hospital Gazette celebrated his disinterrment in *Passim*.

They were followed by the rockets, called the V2, Hitlers second vengeance weapon against London. The last of this phase of bombing was in March 1945.

> There was a lull of about six weeks before the rockets began. At last the Germans had invented a missile against which no precautions whatsoever could be taken. This was a great relief to everyone: there was no more of the ducking and diving under tables that characterised the flying-bomb era.

In charge of the surgical organisation for wartime Guys Hospital was Mr Hedley Atkins, from 1939 until he went to North Africa with the Royal Army Medical Corps (RAMC) in 1942. Russell Brock took care of the chest surgery. His lecture on chest injuries given in August 1945 and published in the *Gazette* reflected the experience he had acquired as a result of the bombardment.[9]

> Fractured ribs and other forms of injury to the chest, quite apart from gunshot wounds, have become much more common as a result of the war; this is due to falling masonry during aerial bombing, and in part the greater incidence of accidents to mechanical vehicles.

Returning to normal

As the war in Europe drew to its end Guys Hospital was returning to normality. Although the war is not the subject of this story, the aftermath of the war fostered an environment in which leadership, risk taking and team work flourished. The medical school staff and preclinical students had been in Tunbridge Wells for the duration. In his capacity as one of the senior physicians, Dr Maurice Campbell left Guys with 87 nurses to set up a hospital in a collection of huts from World War One in Orpington in Kent, about 15 miles out of London.[10] Dr Campbell did not return to Guys until 1946. He was then aged 54 but was soon to embark upon a whole new phase of his career.

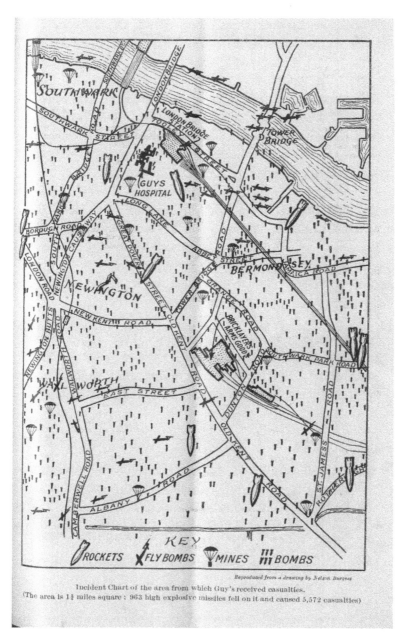

Explosive missiles in Guys casualty receiving
area during World War Two.
Guys Hospital Gazette 1st September 1945.

During the period 1945 to 1948, which this introduction covers, there were external forces that Guys men had to come to terms with in a post-war world. These are reflected in the *Guy's Hospital Gazette*, which was published fortnightly and contained news, comment, correspondence, job adverts, sports and examination results, and full accounts of the regular programme of lectures which were open to all students and staff. One topic was the impending National Health Service.[11] It seems likely that this was an enabling factor in the Peacock Clubs ability to use resources as they strove to develop heart surgery. A bone of contention for some young doctors was the allocation to returning servicemen of training posts usually available to qualifying students. Dr Boland, the Dean who had served through two world wars, losing an eye in the first of them, joined the correspondence to steer it in a more constructive direction.[12] And then, particularly worrying for some was the directive that women students were to be admitted – but the general prevailing view was to at least accept the inevitable.

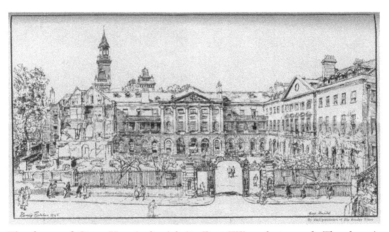

The front of Guys Hospital with its East Wing destroyed. The drawing by Mr Hanslip Fletcher was published in The Times on July 8th 1945. It was reproduced with permission in Guys Hospital Gazette on 1st September 1945 and is reproduced here under licence from The Times. The East Wing was rebuilt as Boland House.

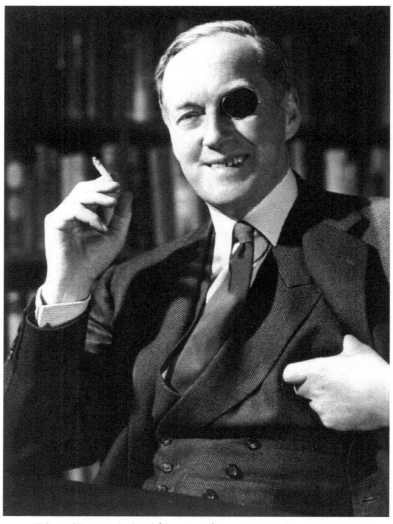

Edward Rowan Boland (1898–1972) Physician at Guys Hospital and Dean of the Medical School (1945–65). Image from the Gordon Museum, Guys. See Biographical Notes for details.

External influences towards heart surgery

Meanwhile two factors specifically affecting thoracic surgery arose from the experience of war. They were instrumental in determining the direction which Maurice Campbell and his surgical colleague Russell Brock would take, encouraging them to embark on a programme of heart operations. One was the practical demonstration by the American surgeon Dwight Harken that the heart was no longer a no go area for surgeons.

In 1944, when he was barely 34 years of age Dr Harken was made head of thoracic surgery in the American armys first designated specialist chest centre.[13] There had been resistance. Dr Elliot Cutler, who was in charge of the American forces medical care in the European Theatre of Operations, believed in the complete surgeon who was prepared to take on anything. Cutler wanted only general hospitals.[13] Harken had worked in the Brompton Hospital with Tudor Edwards, who with his colleagues had been developing thoracic surgery very much as a specialty. Cutler was overruled and General Paul Hawley, the top medical man in the American army, appointed Harken to lead a thoracic surgical service in a hospital shared with neurosurgery. The 160th US General Hospital was another wartime collection of huts erected just outside Cirencester in Gloucestershire. The name General Hospital stuck but the reality was a specialist hospital.

From D-Day on 6 June 1944 there was an influx of soldiers with chest injuries, brought in from France. Many had bullets and shrapnel in their chests and some of the projectiles were within the chambers of the heart or the large adjacent blood vessels. But these soldiers had survived to be brought across the channel with these missiles inside them. There is no imperative to operate to remove a bullet that is not doing any harm simply by being there. So again Harken faced opposition from some surgical seniors, but he set out on a programme of surgery to remove these foreign bodies. Harken had the tacit support of Tudor Edwards who was adviser for thoracic casualties to the Ministry of Health and to the War Office. There was a risk to young Dr Harkens reputation but in the event he removed bullets and shrapnel from the hearts of 56 American soldiers from the 1944 D-Day landings without a death.[14] Russell Brock went twice to Cirencester to watch Harken operating to remove bullets in the heart. Harken presented this surgical experience to the Association of Surgeons of Great Britain and Ireland in May 1945.[14]

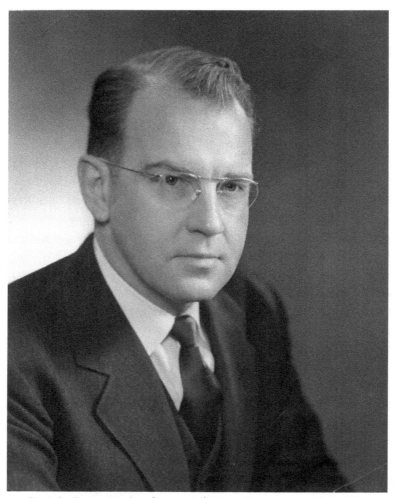

Dwight Emary Harken (1910–1993) Thoracic surgeon at the 160th US General Hospital, Cirencester in Gloucestershire, England at the time of the D-Day landings in 1944. Image from Countway Library, Harvard Medical School. See Biographical Notes for details.

Brock had seen it done and knew that direct operation within the heart was possible. What was more important was that the evidence had been shown to his colleagues, and to the surgical profession as a body, that working inside the hearts was achievable without death due to bleeding, infection, or loss of the hearts rhythm and function.[13]

The Gift of the Company of Clothworkers

A crucial determinant of Brock and Campbell embarking on heart surgery, was the exchange programme with Johns Hopkins that brought to Guys another American, Alfred Blalock.[15] Dr Rowan Boland had served in the army from 1940 at first in a field hospital in the desert campaign in Africa. During 1943 he was at the allied forces headquarters in Sicily with responsibilities to oversee army medical care in North Africa, Italy and Greece, holding the rank of brigadier. His American counterpart there was Perrin Long of Johns Hopkins. It is thought that the encounter sparked the idea of an exchange programme.[*] In August 1946, Dr Boland wrote as the Dean of Guys Hospital Medical School to his opposite number Dr Alan Chesney at Johns Hopkins Hospital, Baltimore with the idea of exchanging clinical teachers with those of an American Hospital.

Bo Boland had a flair for administration which was evident in his wartime service. He was appointed Dean on his return to Guys and soon wrote to Dr Chesney at Johns Hopkins:

> The object of the exchange would be to maintain the friendship, cooperation and exchange of ideas which has been one of the better things which have come out of this War and of which so many of our joint Staffs have so much personal experience ... The Company of Clothworkers, one of our old City Companies, has had the generous imagination to see the value of this proposal and has granted £1,000 per annum for financial expenses this end for at least a number of years.

---

* http://esgweb1.nts.jhu.edu/hmn/S05/annals.cfm
Letter dated 28th August 1946 from Dr Boland to Dr Chesney. AMC Archive, Johns Hopkins

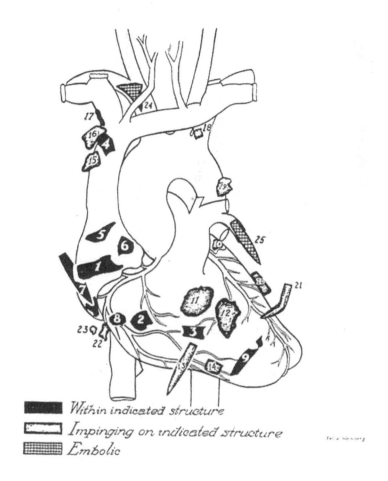

A drawing illustrating 56 missiles and pieces of shrapnel within or impinging on the hearts of soldiers after the D-Day landings of WW2. In total missiles were successfully removed from the chests of 134 soldiers by Dr Harken with no deaths. The illustration and its legend are from Harkens presentation to the Association of Surgeons of Great Britain and Ireland in 1945.[14]

The proposal was accepted with enthusiasm. In January 1947 the arrangement was formalised at the Guys Medical Committee. It was agreed that the representative sent be chosen by the sending hospital and it was decided by Johns Hopkins that Dr Alfred Blalock would be the first to come to Guys. He had by then already achieved remarkable success in dramatically improving the lives of hundreds of blue babies by operation.[13]

Blue babies

So-called blue babies were a familiar sight at the time. Their blueness corresponded to low levels of oxygen in the blood circulating around their bodies: the bluer the child the lower the oxygen saturation and the poorer their stamina. They all had in common some defect that allowed blue blood to reach the bodys circulation. The normally built heart keeps blue and red blood flowing in two completely separate streams, one circulation directing blue blood to the lungs and the other providing oxygenated red blood to the body. However some congenital heart defects involve a hole in the wall between the two sides of the heart and this sabotages the obligatory separation of blue and red blood. The path of least resistance is then for some of the red blood to cross to the more compliant, lower pressure side and go back round the lungs. If there is narrowing or obstruction of the path to the lungs, the blood goes the other way and blue oxygen depleted blood goes around the body.

The standard textbook of medicine, edited by Guys senior physician Sir John Conybeare, told the students: In a large group of cases cyanosis is the first sign and is so characteristic that blue baby and congenital heart disease are practically synonymous.[16] They would also learn that there was nothing to be done about it. There was an obstruction to the flow of blood to lungs and communication between the right and left sides so that most of the blood never reached the lungs and went round the body again without picking up the vital oxygen. Any exertion, crying or feeding increased the need for oxygen and with even less oxygen being delivered to the brain, these children could sporadically lapse into unconsciousness.

Dr Campbell's Lecture, Guy's 1946

In a lecture at Guys on Congenital Heart Disease in January 1946, Maurice Campbell opened by saying Sometimes this seems a dull subject because of the lack of treatment for the condition, so there is a feeling that it does not much matter about the diagnosis.[17] He justified the lecture by explaining that there was value in being able to advise the patients on how much they should do (based on awareness of often how little they could do) and to give a prognosis to the parents. Dr Campbells own experience indicated that of those that survived infancy, about half of the children died before the age of seven, only one in five lived to fourteen, and very few survived to adult life. Closing the notes on his lecture, under the heading Pulmonary Stenosis and Fallots Tetrad Campbell told them I do not intend to say much about the last group on my list because they are the grossly cyanosed cases for which not much in the way of treatment can be done beyond controlling the activities of the patient.[17]

Helen Taussig, Vivien Thomas and Alfred Blalock

Unknown at the time to Maurice Campbell there was a challenge to this received wisdom. At the instigation of the paediatrician Dr Taussig, Blalock devised his operation with laboratory technician Vivien Thomas playing a major role. The surgery was not on the heart itself, but on the arteries close to it. It was a means of diverting some blood back to the lungs where it could be oxygenated. These children were, for the first time in their lives, pink or at least very much less blue than they had been.[18] Blalocks operations were not performed within the heart. They were an indirect means of dealing with the problem but so successful that the results had a major impact on the attitude to surgery for heart disease. Hedley Atkins and Russell Brock who had spent the early part of the war working together at Guys were active and influential committee members as can be seen from papers of Guys Hospital committees at the London Metropolitan Archive. It is likely that they influenced the choice of Alfred Blalock to be the first exchange visitor from Baltimore. The choice was critically important in subsequent events.

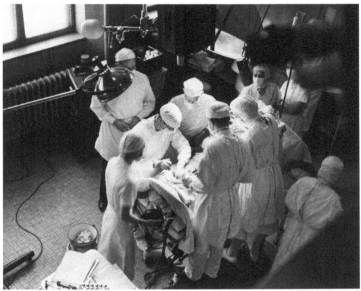

Alfred Blalock operating on a Blue Baby at Johns Hopkins. Vivien Thomas is standing just behind Blalock. Assisting Dr Blalock and standing opposite him is believed to be Denton Cooley and to his left William Longmire. Reproduced with permission from the Alan Mason Chesney Archives of the Johns Hopkins Medical Institutions.

Dr Alfred Blalock exchange visit
Hedley Atkins had just been made director of the newly designated Surgical Department at Guys and it was his prerogative to make plans with the visiting American surgeon. He wrote to Dr Blalock in February 1947:

> When you arrive I shall be responsible for arranging what you would like to do at Guys and I should like to have some preliminary ideas. I have charge of, at the moment, I fear only eleven beds and should you wish I would be delighted to put these eleven beds entirely at your disposal, so that you would have the opportunity of operating ... Of course we are all extremely anxious to see your operation for congenital pulmonary stenosis, and I have sent word round to the Physicians warning them to look out for suitable cases.[*]

---

[*] Letter dated 5th February 1947 from Hedley Atkins to Dr Blalock, AMC Archive, Johns Hopkins.

The Heart Club

We know from Dr Campbells lecture later in the year that he had already started looking for patients since September 1946.[290] Alfred Blalock replied to Hedley Atkins in a long, charming and rather diffident letter. He touched on the English weather, comparing it unfavourably to that of the southern states which he and his wife were accustomed to. He covered matters regarding their travel and accommodation. He wrote that hed had a hectic year and would be willing to take a rest. But the nub of his letter which Hedley Atkins acted upon was this:

> I will, however, be glad to do anything that you wish me to do ... If you think that it will be helpful in any way, I will be glad to operate or assist someone in operating on one or more patients with pulmonic stenosis. I would prefer patients in the age group from 3–8.*

Dr and Mrs Blalock sailed on the Mauritania leaving New York on August 22nd 1947 and stayed at The Norfolk Hotel, Surrey Street, Strand, London from August 29th until September 25th at a cost, including breakfast, of £1.18s per night. Details such as this, found in the Johns Hopkins archives, allow us to appreciate the purchasing power of the Clothmakers £1,000 per annum. The letters to and fro, many of them handwritten, are a mix of collegiality and domesticity. The Blalocks had ordered a parcel of fine food to be sent as gifts to their London hosts but somehow it disappeared en route. Mrs Blalock, tired of corresponding with the shipping company to no avail, left it to her husband but there seems to have been no resolution, at least as far as the Johns Hopkins archives revealed. Apart from that irritation the trip was a resounding success.

Blalocks arrival was announced in the *Gazette* which devoted the whole of *Passim* to welcoming the visitors.[15] The *Gazette* piece concludes:

> An operation performed by Professor Blalock on Tuesday September 2nd on a case of Pulmonary Stenosis was, we believe, the first of its kind to be carried out in this country.

---

* Letter dated March 18th 1947 from Alfred Blalock to Mr Atkins, AMC Archive, Johns Hopkins.

GUY'S HOSPITAL GAZETTE

A Journal of Medicine, Surgery, Dentistry and Hospital News

PUBLISHED FORTNIGHTLY

Vol. LXI. No. 1543   13th September 1947   *Ninepence*

PASSIM

IT is with great pleasure that we welcome to Guy's, Professor Alfred Blalock from the Johns Hopkins Foundation, Baltimore. This eminent surgeon's name is famous throughout the world for his work on the surgical treatment of Congenital Heart Disease and it is indeed a great honour for our hospital to entertain him during his stay in England.

Professor Blalock has, for a short while, left the land of the mighty dollar and entered this austerity island of the frustrated farthing. What will he think of post-war Great Britain in general and, even more to the point, what will he think of Guy's Hospital in particular? All of us on this side of the Atlantic are always assured of at least two things by our American visitors—firstly, of the excellence of our policemen, and secondly, of the horrors of our coffee. What of a British hospital compared with one in the United States?

It is imagined by many of us that all American hospitals are huge, white-stoned edifices somewhat resembling super-cinemas, staffed by sunburnt athletes and nylon-draped glamour girls. Hollywood, in best scientific manner, goes further still and gives the impression that everyone is either " starting the Adrenaline," " stopping the Adrenaline," or " preparing a hypodermic," whilst every operation is performed by a sort of immaculately dressed cricket team and is such a dramatic procedure that even the theatre sister's mascara runs.

Fortunately this description is just so much celluloid fantasy and already we have learnt from Mr. Eckhoff some of his impressions of American surgery and the ways in which their policy differs from ours.

One visitor to our hospital recently described it as " quaint and interesting." The matter was not pursued further, but we flatter ourselves that the quaintness referred to some of our architectural structures and not to our clinical methods, as our visitor, to the best of our knowledge, was not shown any cases that had been either cupped, leeched, or touched for the King's Evil. Nevertheless we must admit that the radiance of Dorcas does contrast *quaintly* with the shadows of Ruth where physical signs lie engulfed in never-ending gloom. Similarly the intermittent outbursts of Works Department Artillery must doubtless make *quaint* music to the unaccustomed ear, and the even *quainter* grumblings of our few functioning lifts can strike terror in the stoutest of hearts, be they of oak or American pine.

During his stay we are sure that Professor Blalock will be able to teach us much of American cardiac surgery and as we understand that the " blue baby " waiting list at Guy's is steadily increasing, it would seem that many of us may have the privilege of witnessing this new kind of operative technique.

On 13th September 1947 Guys Hospital Gazette
published this warm welcome to Alfred Blalock.

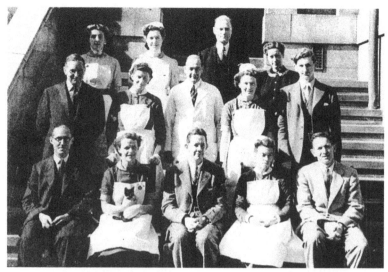

A group photograph on the steps of Guys Hospital Medical School September 1947. Back row: Staff nurse, Staff nurse, Hedley Atkins, Matron Dorothy M Smith. Middle: Dr Rink, Sister, Kenneth Allanby, Staff nurse, Brian McEvedy. Front: Russell Brock, Sister, Alfred Blalock, Sister Fallwasser, Henry Bahnson

Blalock performed ten of his subclavian to pulmonary artery operations; there were no deaths. The visit featured in the national and regional newspapers.

The International Conference of Physicians
Blalocks visit included much more besides operating. His visit was scheduled to include attendance at the International Conference of Physicians which met in London on 8th and 9th September 1947. The meeting was reported in both the *BMJ* and *The Lancet*.[20;21] With four to five hundred physicians attending the outstanding event of the conference on Sept. 9 was an all-day discussion on the surgery of congenital heart disease, for which the Sections of Paediatrics and Cardiology combined.[21] Helen Taussig and Alfred Blalock were the opening speakers and were much praised for their work. Tubbs and Crafoord, noted for their contributions on the surgery of patent ductus arteriosus and coarctation, were prominent among the speakers.[22;23] The conference was written up at length in the *British Heart Journal*.[24]

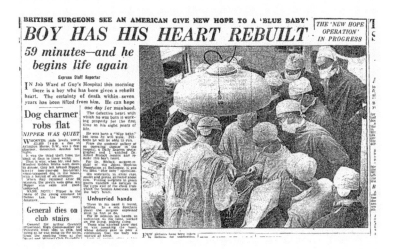

The Daily Express on Monday 15 September 1947 reported one of the early operations by Alfred Blalock at Guys Hospital. The description of the operation is inaccurate but the picture captures the rapt attention of those present. The surgeon whose hands can be seen operating is Blalock. Opposite him and with his back to us is the tall figure of Henry Bahnson. The man leaning forward (with his nose above his mask) is Russell Brock. Reproduced with permission from the Daily Express.

As intended by the exchange arrangement, Blalock gave lectures and demonstrations, and contributed generally to the teaching of the Hospital, as well as operating. Within a packed schedule Hedley Atkins announced in the *Gazette* that on Saturday 13th September Dr Blalock would conduct a departmental round in Queen Ward and on Friday 19th September there would be a visit of the International Congress of Surgeons to Guys.[25] Blalock gave the Moynihan Lecture at the Royal College of Surgeons on 26th September.[26] Soon after Drs Blalock and Bahnson went on to Paris to do more blue baby operations and then flew home, with their wives, via Shannon on 13th October 1947.

TETRALOGY OF FALLOT

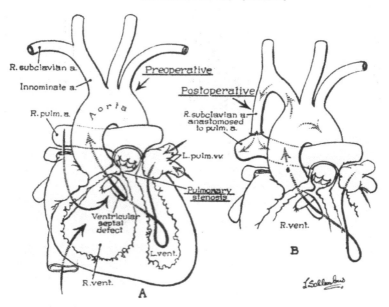

Fig. 1A. Diagram showing the tetralogy of Fallot. This demonstrates the pulmonic stenosis in the conus region, the interventricular septal defect, the aorta which overrides the defect and receives some venous blood, and the right venticular hypertrophy.

Fig. 1B. Diagram showing the tetralogy of Fallot after operation. The proximal end of the right subclavian artery has been anastomosed to the side of the right pulmonary artery, thus shunting incompletely oxygenated blood from the aorta into the pulmonary arteries.

These drawings and their original captions are from the Moynihan Lecture given by Alfred Blalock on 26th September 1947 during his exchange visit to Guys. It was published in the Annals of the Royal College of Surgeons of England in 1948. [26]

In November Maurice Campbell wrote to Blalock saying the patients are accumulating at a faster rate than we can deal with them and hoped that Blalock would have no objection to him writing up progress reports for publication. The details of these and subsequent operations by the Guys team were written up in *Guy's Hospital Reports* [19] and later in the *BMJ* after 200 operations had been completed.[28] Subsequent correspondence which I was privileged to read in the Johns Hopkins archives indicates great warmth and enthusiasm at a personal level, with Brock, Campbell and Atkins continuing to correspond with Blalock.

Dr Maurice Campbell's revised attitude to cyanotic heart disease

On October 1947, after Blalock had returned to Baltimore, Campbell lectured again and this time the title was Cyanosis and Morbus Cruleus [290]: it was specifically about cyanotic congenital heart disease.

> In January 1946, when I came back after the war I gave a lecture on congenital heart disease; there had been considerable progress as regards patent ductus arteriosus and coarctation but I am sorry to say that I dismissed cyanotic heart disease in the last two paragraphs of my lecture because I said there was nothing to be done for it.[290]

Campbells reflections on the dramatic results of surgery are worth quoting at some length.

> ...a few words about the actual results in these cases. Many of you have seen them in the wards and observed the improvement while they were there. Last week I saw the first three back at the hospital for the first time since they had been discharged. I was almost alarmed at the amount they were doing. ... I did not appreciate how much a child, suddenly relieved of his lifelong disability might want to do. From the parents point of view these three are cured children who are leading normal lives. One of them who had rarely walked more than about 10 yards is now running about all day; the parents say it is very difficult to stop him doing anything.[290]

A *Daily Express* photographer had taken a picture of this three year old boy named Peter, the third of the Guys patients to be operated on by Blalock.[19] The celebrated portrait photographer Yousuf Karsh pictured Blalock putting Peters framed picture up on the wall in Baltimore. In the well-known picture of Blalock smoking (as most men did at that time) there is a smaller framed version of Peters picture next to him. That fabulous picture of Blalock hangs in pride of place in the Johns Hopkins archive reading room. The archivist told me that she had been looking at that picture for 30 years and never made the connection. There is something remarkable, that after as many as 500 blue babies treated, that this little boy should have made his way onto the surgeons office wall in Johns Hopkins and into Yousuf Karshs portrait.

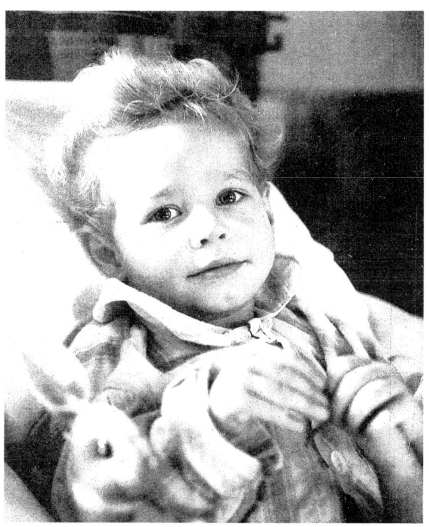

This little boy called Peter was the third child to be operated on during Alfred Blalocks visit to Guys.[19] He received special personal mention in Maurice Campbells lecture to Guys students on 31st October 1947.[290] The photograph was copied for me by the Alan Mason Chesney Archives of the Johns Hopkins Medical Institutions with the permission of Express Newspapers.

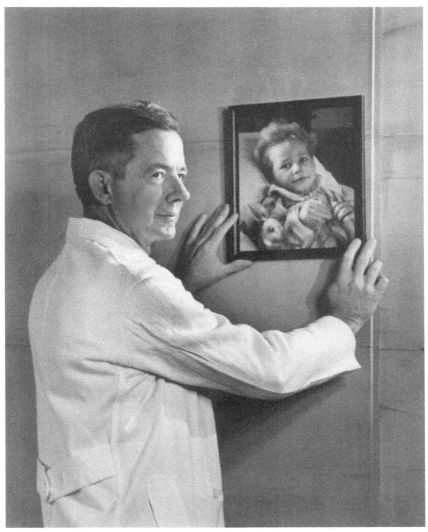

Dr Alfred Blalock, back home in Baltimore put the framed picture of Peter on the wall of his department in Johns Hopkins Hospital. Picture from the Estate of Yousuf Karsh.

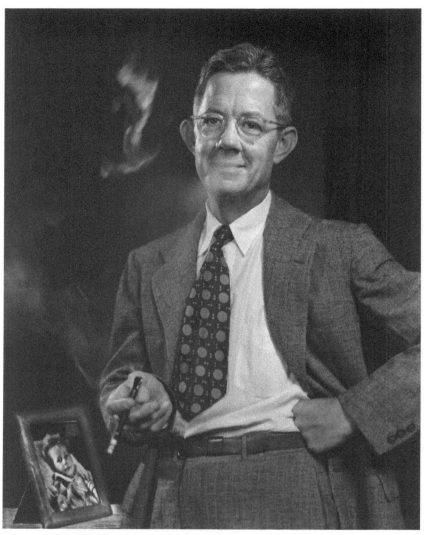

Alfred Blalock 1950
Image provided by the Estate of Yousuf Karsh

Fallot's Tetralogy: the relative importance of the ventricular septal defect and pulmonary stenosis

The success of Blalocks surgery in improving cyanosis and the stamina of these children settled one matter of debate. Sceptics reasonably took the view that while there was a large ventricular septal defect that could not be repaired, that bypassing the pulmonary stenosis with Blalocks operation would not make enough difference to make it worthwhile. But now the empirical evidence was there: the shunt gave benefit in most cases and a big difference in many. So if bypassing the stenosis could achieve a worthwhile improvement, why not a direct approach on the stenosis? Here we see the importance of Harkens influence. Maurice Campbell had written in his lecture after Blalocks visit *all this time Mr Brock had been discussing with me a more direct attack on pulmonary stenosis* [290] so Campbell was open to the idea. Both Sellors and Brock had relieved pulmonary stenosis by direct operations on the valve in 1947 and 1948. These operations were reported in *The Lancet* and the *BMJ* respectively.[29;30] There was a question of precedence but there is no reason to think it was a bone of contention. Thomas Holmes Sellors was referred to by one and all as Uncle Tom for good reason – he was an amiable man. As to the facts of the matter, I researched the dates with Dr Arthur Hollman 50 years after the events and we concluded that Thomas Holmes Sellors should rightly be attributed the first; but Brock had written up his three cases before Holmes Sellors got into print.[31]

Surgery for mitral stenosis

Mitral stenosis very soon became part of the work of the Peacock Club so I will introduce some background here. For 50 years there had been sporadic suggestions that mitral stenosis might be relieved by surgery. Daniel West Samways examined reports of 4,791 necropsies on patients dying in Guys Hospital from 1886 to 1895 and identified 196 cases whom he judged on the measurements to have mitral stenosis.[32] In 1898 he wrote in The Lancet *I anticipate that with the progress of cardiac surgery some of the severest cases will be relieved.*[33] A few years later Sir Lauder Brunton wrote in The Lancet a preliminary note.

> Mitral stenosis is not only one of the most distressing forms of cardiac disease, but in its severe form it resists all treatment by medicine.

> On looking at the contracted mitral valve orifice in a severe case of this disease, one is impressed by the hopelessness of ever finding a remedy which will enable the auricle to drive the blood in a sufficient stream through the small mitral orifice, and the wish unconsciously arises that one could divide the constriction as easily during life as one can after death.[34]

This drew mixed attention in the correspondence columns but was put down by the editor.[35] There followed some experimental work but no operations on patients in England until Henry Souttar did his one and only operation on the mitral valve with apparent success in 1925, writing:

> The simplest valvular lesion for surgical interference is stenosis of one of the valves, and of these the mitral valve is perhaps the most accessible ... the relief of the lesions themselves would undoubtedly be of immense service to the patient and must be followed by marked improvement in the general condition.[36]

The patient Lilian Hine became quite a celebrity.[37;38] Souttars was one of ten reported operations performed for mitral stenosis during the 1920s, seven of them by Elliot Cutler. His first appeared to be successful but the next six patients died soon after surgery, four within 24 hours and the other two within a few days. This experience resulted in a paper titled Present status of surgical procedures in chronic valvular disease of the heart; final report of all surgical cases.[39] This was the memory of failed operations within the heart that Harkens success removing bullets and shrapnel helped to dispel.[13;14]

There had been shifting emphasis away from a mechanistic to a holistic perception of the heart in the interwar years.[40] This was influenced by Sir James Mackenzie who set out his stall in three long *BMJ* papers in 1924.[41-43] Cutlers disastrous experience added empirical evidence, bolstering the views of those fundamentally opposed to a mechanistic view of the heart and therefore to surgery as a solution to its ailments. In 1923 Mackenzie had written to Cutlers cardiologist and co-author Dr Sam Levine,[44] Dear Sam, What a foolish thing to try to do. Have you forgotten that the myocardium is all important?[45] Maurice Campbell was a practicing physician in 1923 with MRCP, MD after his name. He was made FRCP in the year Cutler wrote his final report.

Hearsay evidence is that Campbell shared Brocks view that mitral valvotomy might be revisited[46] but they both knew the prevailing view. A representative statement of opinion is this in 1943 from Sir Thomas Lewis:

> Surgical attempts to relieve cases of mitral stenosis ... by cutting the valve have so far failed to give benefit. I think they will continue to fail, not only because the interference is too drastic, but because the attempt is based on what, usually at all events, is an erroneous idea, namely that the valve is the chief source of the problem.[47]

No explicit intent to operate on mitral stenosis by Brock or Campbell was evident in any of the written material I have studied but events within months of the start of the Peacock Club indicate that it cannot have been far from their minds. There was also activity across the Atlantic. In 1945 Charles Bailey began a series of operations but had four deaths in succession.[48] In Boston, Harken had already operated on his first case of mitral stenosis in March 1947 but his patient also died.[49] The five failed operations were not reported until later, when both surgeons had a single success to report, but they were likely to have been known to Brock and were reasons to be cautious.

In 1948 Russell Brock summed up the surgical appeal of dealing with a stenosed valve.

> When one examines the heart post mortem in patients dying of valvular disease and contemplates the minute size of the orifice through which the whole life blood of the body has to be forced it is impossible not to feel that this simple mechanical obstruction must be capable of relief by surgery.[30]

This restates the sentiments of Dr DW Samways, Sir Lauder Brunton and Henry Souttar. Note that this was in the context of surgery for cyanotic heart disease and operations on the pulmonary valve. Mitral stenosis was not mentioned but this was a general statement that might apply to any heart valve: the whole life blood of the body must pass through each in turn and they may be similarly capable of relief by surgery. As we have seen, with respect to mitral stenosis the prevailing view at the time was that it would make no difference; the rheumatic disease had damaged the heart muscle and that was the cause of the patients functional limitation. It was not an auspicious time to tackle the problem of the mitral valve; this was not a cause to take up as they began to build their team to look after blue babies. There were now many patients with cyanotic heart disease being referred and there was a lot of work to be done.

Building capacity
In October 1947 Guys Hospital medical committee agreed to recommend that a Thoracic Surgical Unit should be formed ... under the charge of Mr Brock. In November 1947 Dr Maurice Campbell gave up being a Full Physician to work solely as a cardiologist to deal with the large number of congenital heart disease patients coming to the hospital. The *Gazette* carried adverts for junior doctors to expand the cardiology and thoracic surgery clinical and research staff. By 1948 Guys had a medical and surgical infrastructure in place ready to practise and develop heart surgery.

The Residents' Play
Evidence that Guys was recovering from the war was the return of the residents play which was on stage from 27th to 30th April 1948 the week after the first meeting of the Club. The *Gazette* published a review written by the surgeon Sam Wass.[50]

> This years play, Block Dissection or Why is my Baby so Blue tonight has an amusingly topical plot. The principal character, Mr Block, was engaged on the epoch-making surgical adventure of making red babies blue. This change in colour of the youth of the nation was against the political interest of a group of Reds who were working in the Hospital under orders direct from Moscow.

This follows a generic plot device of Guys residents plays! A group of baddies are trying to take over Guys but the goodies prevail and save the Hospital, in the course of which senior consultants can be parodied. Here, Mr Block came through in the end. Blue baby operations were still newsworthy but sufficiently well established to have become the subject of light-hearted fun. The play was co-written by John Trounce who was on stage alongside John Baylis and Ian Kelsey Fry. They were all to feature in the Peacock Club. Brian McEvedy, who was Brocks houseman during the Blalock visit was also on stage. For Mr Block and his work to provide the plot line, and for him to be the leader of the goodies, was a measure of Brocks standing as a figure in his hospital.

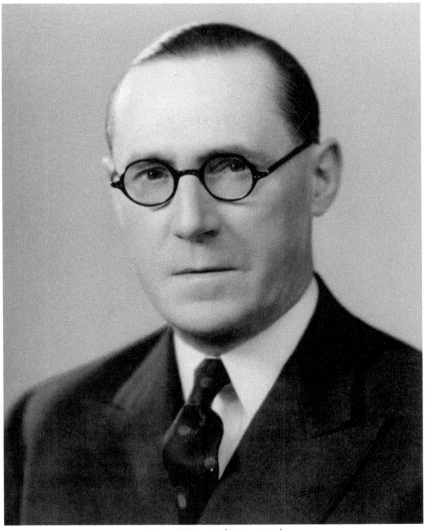

Russell Brock (1903–1980)

PEACOCK
CLUB
—
21 4 48
12 3 56

The Minutes of the Peacock Club 1948–1956

1.	April	1948	Meeting convened and plans made
2.	June	1948	Record keeping, clinical rounds, and referrals discussed
3.	July	1948	Thrombosis, embolism and polycythaemia
4.	September	1948	Clinical cases: preparation for operations on mitral stenosis
5.	November	1948	Dr Campbells analysis of 460 congenital heart patients
6.	December	1948	Angiocardiograms reviewed
7.	January	1949	Professors Willis and Foxon: development of the heart
8.	March	1949	Review of completed cases
9.	April	1949	Dr Holling, the Bing test and heart catheterisation
10.	May	1949	Dr Frances Gardener demonstrated angiocardiography
11.	June	1949	Mr Brock talked about the infundibulum
12.	September	1949	Clinical cases: angiocardiograms and post mortem hearts
13.	November	1949	Clinical cases: angiocardiograms and post mortem hearts
14.	December	1949	Mr Ian Hill on angiocardiograms
15.	February	1950	Mr Brocks American visit
16.	March	1950	Dr Campbell: follow up of cases of direct cardiac operations
17.	April	1950	Dr Brintons paper on the blood before and after operations
18.	September	1950	Surgeons Cooley, ONeill (USA), Barrett, Cleland (London)

The Heart Club

19.	November	1950	Dr Reynolds and Dr Baker on arrhythmias during interventions
20.	January	1951	Dr Holling investigation of patients with mitral stenosis
21.	February	1951	Dr Campbell radiology, blood pressure and blood flow
22.	March	1951	Dr Tom Hills: Fairchild camera and selective angiocardiograms
23.	April	1951	Mr Brock and Dr Trounce: surgical films and pathology
24.	May	1951	Dr Baker on 200 cases of mitral stenosis
25.	July	1951	Dr McMillan showed films of heart valves in action Dr Reynolds paper on the ECG during angiocardiograms
26.	October	1951	Dr Verel on pressure measurements during mitral valvotomy
27.	November	1951	Mr Ian Hill spoke on 162 angiocardiographies
28.	January	1952	Mr Brock on the rheumatic mitral valve
29.	February	1952	Dr Deuchar: cardiovascular pressure in congenital heart disease
30.	March	1952	Drs Baker and Bywaters: acute rheumatism and mitral stenosis
31.	October	1952	Dr Brunner described his experimental work on aortic grafting
32.	November	1952	Dr Enticknap presented lung histology in mitral stenosis Dr Baker showed x-rays of the lungs in mitral stenosis
33.	January	1953	Dr Campbell: natural history of congenital heart disease
34.	February	1953	Dr McMillan: films of heart valve movements
35.	March	1953	Dr Tom Hills: angiocardiograms of special congenital cases
36.	November	1953	Dr Holling reported on his visit to the USA
37.	December	1953	Mr Ross: experiments with hypothermia in dogs
38.	February	1954	Mr Milstein spoke on ventricular fibrillation

39.	March	1954	Dr Shephard: blood flow and pressure with left to right shunt
			Dr Venner and Dr Holling: pressures across the mitral valve
40.	May	1954	Mr Brock: aortic stenosis
41.	December	1954	International Cardiological Congress, Washington
42.	January	1955	Dr Baker: late results of mitral valvotomy
43.	February	1955	Coarctation of the Aorta
44.	March	1955	Sir Russell Brock on recent developments in the USA
45.	December	1955	Dr Campbell and Sir Russell Brock: aortic stenosis
46.	January	1956	Drs Campbell and Brotmacher: ventricular septal defect
47.	March	1956	Drs Catherine Neil, Suzman and Campbell: ASD

The Heart Club

1

A meeting, convened by Mr Brock, of those concerned
in the management of Congenital disease of the Heart, took
place at Guy's Hospital on Wednesday 21 April 1948.
There were present :-
Mr Brock. Dr Charles Baker. Dr Syzman. Dr Holling
Dr Rink. Dr Zak. Mr Hill. Dr Brinton. Dr Channel.
Dr Allanby. Mr Kelsey Fry.

It was proposed by Dr Baker, seconded by Dr Holling,
that Mr Brock should take the chair.

Mr Brock explained his reasons for convening this
meeting under the following heads :-
1. Regular meetings of this kind would enable each
   department in this field to know how work of the other
   departments was proceeding. Meetings to occur monthly.
2. A review of the past months work to be given, and
   a discussion of the next months work to follow, with
   consideration of the state of the waiting - list.
3. Discussion of special investigations ; their apparatus
   and technique.

The first page of the minutes in April 1948. The writer is unknown
and there are no other minutes in this handwriting. The original
volume of the minutes has been placed in the Arthur Hollman
Collection of the British Cardiovascular Society. A full sequence
of facsimiles made by the present author is available as .jpg files.

April 1948

A meeting, convened by Mr Brock,* of those concerned in the management of Congenital disease of the Heart, took place at Guys Hospital on Wednesday 21 April 1948.

There were present:
Mr Brock, Dr Charles Baker, Dr Suzman, Dr Holling, Dr Rink, Dr Zak, Mr Hill, Dr Brinton, Dr Channell, Dr Allanby,§ Mr Kelsey Fry.¶

It was proposed by Dr Baker, seconded by Dr Holling, that Mr Brock should take the chair.

Mr Brock explained his reasons for convening this meeting under the following heads:

1. Regular meetings of this kind would enable each department in this field to know how work of the other departments was proceeding. Meetings to occur monthly.
2. A review of the past months work to be given, and a discussion of the next months work to follow, with consideration of the state of the waiting list.
3. Discussion of special investigations; their apparatus and technique.
4. There should be a Central Register of patients, whereby admissions for investigation and operation could be organised. Various systems of indexing were suggested, chiefly the punch-card system.** It was agreed

---

* It remains British custom for doctors who train as surgeons to drop the title Dr and revert to Mr. A reminder is Barber-Surgeons Hall in Monkwell Square in London. Surgeons are qualified medical doctors with a general training and later specialise in surgery.

 Variously spelled with s or ss but I am confident of this spelling and the identification.

 Sometimes spelled Channel but the identity is secure from publications and there is no reasonable alternative to Dr Channell.

§ Sometimes Allenby but I am confident of the identity being Allanby as in the Biographical Notes.

¶ We believe this was Ian Kelsey Fry who was Brocks houseman. His father was also at Guys and both are listed in the Biographical Notes.

** See punch-card system in the Glossary.

The Heart Club

that members should inform the secretaries of the headings under which patients should be classified.

5. That appropriate journals should be covered by members in the manner of the Journal Club. Also that a reprint library should be accumulated.

6. That part of each meeting be devoted to the discussion of a particular problem. It was agreed that at the next meeting the haematological side of cyanotic* heart disease be discussed, with special reference to thrombosis, and that Dr Waterfield and Dr McArdle be invited to be present. Also resolved that the joint secretaries should prepare notes of such cases as had exhibited intravascular thrombosis.

7. That at each meeting there be a pathological discussion with demonstration of recent material by Dr Allanby.

8. That a weekly round should take place attended by members of this meeting, for the purpose of securing clinical correlation between the medical and surgical aspects of the problems of Congenital Heart Disease. After discussion as to whether these rounds could be combined with ordinary teaching rounds, it was agreed they were better held separately, and the time of 5pm every Friday was agreed on, the first to take place on Friday 23 April 1948.

Dr Baker proposed that more copies of notes be made since the frequent loss of a single master-copy led to much confusion. He suggested that at least enough copies should be made to necessitate the use of a reproducing method other than carbon copies from a single typewriter (20 copies suggested). He further suggested that the Medical School Office be approached as to whether their machine could be used.

He also explained the functions of the secretary of the Cardiological department, and observed that she also served the Haematological department. It was suggested that this secretary should be employed to keep the Central Registry above-mentioned.

---

* See cyanotic in the Glossary.

The Guys cardiac surgeons had a joint round on Friday afternoons 1970–71 when I was the house surgeon and this was sometimes followed by an academic or research meeting. I never heard of the Peacock Club until I saw the rediscovered book of the Minutes.

Tom Treasure

Dr Brinton proposed that some method be used to impress on the home doctor of cases sent up to Guys, the necessity of PMs should they die outside the hospital. This could be either a special proforma included in the letter to the doctor after the case had been first seen, or some formula in the final paragraph of this letter.

Dr Baker said he had been considering this on a wider basis, and suggested that all cases likely to provide important PM material should be given a special card which would give them ready entry into the hospital. It was agreed between Dr Baker and Mr Brock that this matter would be taken up in an appropriate committee.

Dr Allanby offered to do PMs on cases dying at home and suggested that the general practitioners be informed that this service is available.

The case of the patient HART was then described; before, during and after operations, by Dr Allanby, Mr Brock and Dr Rink. The heart was then shown by Dr Allanby.

The meeting finished with a vote of thanks to Mr Brock for the excellent dinner provided.

June 9th 1948. Maurice Campbell

The Heart Club

5

> Minutes of a meeting of those concerned in the management of cases of Congenital Morbus Cordis held on Wednesday 9th June 1948 at Guys Hospital
>
> There were present
> D' Campbell, chairman; M' Brock, D' Baker D' Suzman, D' Allenby, D' Channel, D' Zak M' Hill · M' Earl.
>
> ① The minutes of the previous meeting were read + approved.
> ② D' Campbell raised the question of a name for the gathering + after suggestions of "The True Blues" + the "Peacock Club" it was decided that the final decision be deferred.
> ③ The question of the proforma to be used in an endeavour to secure autopsies on cases dying outside the hospital was discussed it was agreed that M' Brock + D' Campbell would arrange a draft.
> ④ D' Allenby volunteered to establish a travelling P.M. service + the question of the distance over which this might have to operate was mentioned

The first page of the minutes of the second meeting in June 1948. The handwriting is that of Mr Ian Hill. The naming of the Club is discussed and the decision was deferred.

Tom Treasure

June 1948

Minutes of a meeting of those concerned in the management of cases of Congenital Morbus Cordis*. Held on Wednesday 9th June 1948 at Guys Hospital.

There were present:
Dr Campbell, chairman; Mr Brock, Dr Baker, Dr Suzman, Dr Allanby, Dr Channell, Dr Zak, Mr Hill, Mr Earl.

1. The minutes of the previous meeting were read & approved.
2. Dr Campbell raised the suggestion of a name for the gathering and after suggestions of The True Blues & the Peacock Club but it was decided that the final decision be deferred.
3. The question of the pro forma to be used in an endeavour to secure autopsies on cases dying outside the hospital was discussed and it was agreed that Mr Brock and Dr Campbell would arrange a draft.
4. Dr Allanby volunteered to establish a travelling PM service, the question of the distance over which this might have to operate was mentioned.
5. Mr Brock then opened a discussion on record keeping, observing that many case notes appeared not to be available from the central registry. On the subject of duplicating, whilst Dr Baker has suggested 20 copies of notes, it seemed that only four were essential viz for Hospital Central Registry; Cardiac Unit (Medical), Thoracic Surgical Unit; and Outpatient department. Mr Brock stated that a room would shortly be available for the Surgical Thoracic Unit that he thought that though separate surgical Chest records would be kept, the main cardiac records should be medical and that these should be furnished with surgical reports on those undergoing surgery.
6. Mr Brock proposed that lists should be maintained of cardiac cases (a) investigated and awaiting operation and (b) of those awaiting investigation.
7. Dr Campbell inquired what number of cardiac catheterisations would be completed each week and Dr Zak stated that the present methods the capacity of the department was two per week. In view of this it was decided that cases should be arranged in order of priority (possibly on the Friday rounds) by Drs Holling and Baker.

---

* See Glossary for congenital morbus cordis.
  See cardiac catheterisation in the Glossary.

The Heart Club

8. Arrangements for *angiocardiography were made, the programme for the next week discussed. It was agreed that the most simple routine would be for the H.P. in charge of cases for angiocardiography to contact Mr Hill who would make the final arrangement with the x-ray department.

   The relative values of catheterisation and angiocardiography were discussed and the risks indicated by mishaps reported from the literature.

9. It was next decided that Friday was the most inconvenient day for the combined cardiac round; but that Monday would be a more suitable day for the monthly meeting.

   Dr Channell proposed that there was much to recommend the first Monday in each month and accordingly July 5th was fixed as the date for the next meeting, when the subject of thrombosis would be discussed. It was suggested that Dr McArdle and Dr Waterfield be invited to be present.

10. The case of Doris Savigar was then recorded and the significance of low arterial oxygen saturation and shunt were discussed together with the mitral stenotic element. Dr Allenby suggested the pulmonary factor was a significant one in the production of cyanosis.

11. *

12. The use of Bings test came under discussion and Dr Campbell gave some reflections on the mass of material accumulated in America by the methods of cardiac catheterisation.

13. Dr Allanby then shewed the specimens in the complete cases§ of Doris Savigar & Marian Cox in which connexion the question of laparoscopy¶ to determine cirrhosis of the liver** was raised.

14. The meeting was closed at 11.15 pm with a vote of thanks to Dr Campbell for the excellent dinner at the George.

Maurice Campbell
12.7.48

---

* See angiocardiography in the Glossary.

 Ian Hill maintained his commitment to angiocardiography and appears to have done a large proportion of the interventional part of the work.[51]

 Dr Campbell had recently returned from a visit to Johns Hopkins from where Bing and colleagues had contributed several papers on the subject.[52-55]

§ See complete cases in the Glossary.

¶ See laparoscopy in the Glossary.

** See cirrhosis of the liver in the Glossary.

Minutes of a meeting of those concerned in the management of cases of Congenital Morbus Cordis held on ~~Wednesday~~ Monday 12ᵗʰ July 1948

There were present :——
D Campbell in the chair + Mr Brock, D Baker D Meadle
D Wakefield D Suzman D Rink D Hollup D Zak
D Channel D Brinton Mr Hill + Mr Earl.

The minutes of the last meeting were read + approved

D Campbell quoted from the work of Peacock in 1858 + proposed from the chair that the name "Peacock Club" be adopted. This was seconded by D Bake + Mr Brock + carried nem. com.

The autopsy request form draft + readmission request for heart cases was read + approved

Mr Brock reported the laparoscopy findings on the case of Bradshaw.

The discussion on Thrombosis was then introduced by Mr Brock. D Suzman described 4 cases of cerebral thrombosis in 200 outpatients with

The third meeting of the Club in July 1948 during which the name Peacock Club was decided.

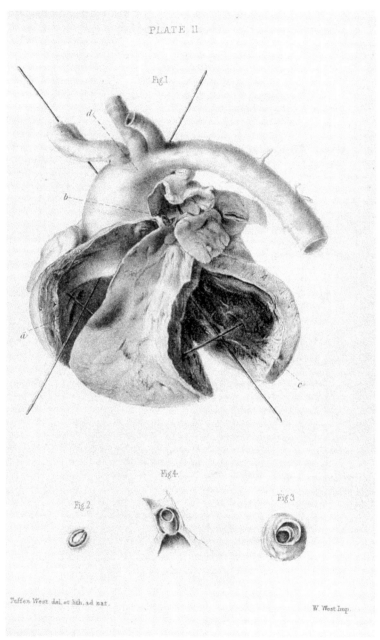

From *On malformations, &c., of the human heart: with original cases* (1858) by Thomas Peacock.[2]

Tom Treasure

Plate 2.—Obstruction at the Orifice of the Pulmonary Artery, and defect in the Septum Ventriculorum.

Fig. 1. Drawing of the heart described at p. 36.

The preparation is marked B 4, in the Museum of the Victoria Park Hospital. The child was 2 years and 5 months old.

a. The right ventricle laid open.

b. The contracted aperture of the pulmonary artery.

c. The left ventricle.

d. The ascending aorta.

The bristles passed into the aorta from behind and visible above the upper edge of the vessel, are seen to pass into both ventricles.

Fig. 2. Form of the valves of the pulmonary artery in this specimen.

Figs. 3 and 4 display the form of the valvular apparatus in the case of Mr. Marshall, described at p. 41.

The preparation is numbered B 6 in the Museum of the Victoria Park Hospital. The boy who was the subject of this malformation was 6½ years of age.

Fig. 3 exhibits the valves as seen from above, or from the pulmonary artery.

Fig. 4, with the coats supposed to be divided so as to show, the peculiar infundibular or barrel-shaped aperture from the ventricle into the artery.

From *On malformations, &c.,* of the human heart: with original cases (1858) by Thomas Peacock.[2]

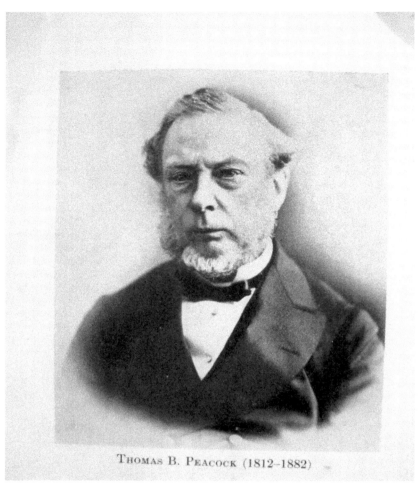

Thomas Peacock (1812–1882)

Tom Treasure

July 1948
Minutes of a meeting of those concerned in the management of cases of
Congenital Morbus Cordis held on Monday 12 July 1948

There were present:
Dr Campbell in the chair & Mr Brock, Dr Baker, Dr McArdle, Dr Waterfield,
Dr Suzman, Dr Rink, Dr Holling, Dr Zak, Dr Channell, Dr Brinton, Mr Hill
and Mr Earl.

1. The minutes of the last meeting were read & approved.
2. Dr Campbell noted from the work of Peacock in 1858 proposed from
    the chair that the name Peacock Club be adopted. This was seconded
    by Dr Baker and Mr Brock and carried *nem con*.
3. The autopsy request form draft and readmission request for heart cases
    was read and approved.
4. Mr Brock reported the laparoscopy findings in the case of Bradshaw.

The discussion on thrombosis was then introduced by Mr Brock. Dr
Suzman described four cases of cerebral thrombosis[*] in 200 outpatients
with congenital heart disease and Mr Hill then gave the records of the five
postoperative thromboses occurring in the 52 cases undergoing operation.

Dr McArdle observed that he favoured paradoxical embolus rather than
thrombosis in these particular cases; noted the high frequency of embolus
in the branches of the vertebral artery and suggested that particular attention should be directed to these vessels at autopsy. He also remarked on the
increased incidence of cerebral venous thrombosis.

Dr Waterfield pointed out that the causal viscosity & slowing was due to
the polycythaemia. At operation the platelet count rose (giving a condition
then comparable with polycythaemia rubra vera)[§] the blood pressure fell
and the fibrinogen content rose. All these factors favoured thrombosis. He
suggested that to combat the condition (i) the viscosity could be reduced by

---

[*] See cerebral thrombosis in the Glossary.
See Glossary for paradoxical embolus.
See platelet count in the Glossary.
[§] See Glossary for polycythaemia.

49

The Heart Club

bleeding[*] (ii) the blood volume, thus B.P., maintained by intravenous plasma or from saline infusion (iii) adequate fluid-intake assured. He felt that the icterus rate with plasma made gum acacia preferable and that the risks of haemorrhage and slow healing associated with the heparin and dicoumarol[§] therapy outweighed the advantage gained. This regime, it was claimed would produce a more rapid return towards a normal haematological picture. Dr Campbell noted that the fall in polycythaemia after operation was more rapid than would be accounted for by red cell death & it was decided to study this process by day to day postoperative blood pictures.

Dr Rink spoke on the question of fluid replacement and did not feel that fall in pressure was a suitable index of blood loss. Fluid replacement estimations were at present empirical; but as a whole he felt error was on the side of underhydration.

Swab weighing and patient weighing were discussed as possible methods of estimating fluid loss and it was finally decided that intake and output charts were the most practical method of assessing dehydration.

Dr Waterfield revised the question of giving iron over a period of months preoperatively to raise the colour index as in cases of polycythaemia rubra vera and it was agreed that control outpatient investigation should be undertaken.

The date of the next meeting was provisionally fixed for 13th September 1948. The meeting was concluded at 10.55 pm.

Sept 13th 1948 Maurice Campbell

---

[*] See bleeding in the Glossary.
See icterus in the Glossary.
See Glossary for gum acacia.
§ See Glossary for dicoumarol.

Tom Treasure

September 1948
Minutes of a meeting of the Peacock Club held on Monday 13th September 1948.

There were present:
Dr Campbell in the chair; Dr Baker, Dr Brock, Dr Tom Hills, Dr Rink, Dr Holling, Dr Zak, Dr Suzman, Dr Brinton, Dr Allanby, Mr Channell, Mr Hill and Mr Hunter.

1. Angiocardiograms of the following cases were demonstrated by Dr Hills and the significant findings discussed: Raymond Sharp, John Chapman, Edward Turner, Mary Stewart, Rita Whalley, Jean May, Mrs Metcalfe, Valerie Farmer, K Simpson and Doris Sawyer.
2. The minutes of the last meeting were read and approved.
3. The proposed operation on Mary Stewart was discussed and a decision made on a preoperative venesection* of 1 pt on the day before.
4. The question of an adequately sensitive man balance was again raised and the possibility of obtaining one from a commercial firm noted.
5. Dr Zak presented the cardiac catheterisation report on Doris Diggins (Mitral Stenosis).
   The policy of refraining from angiocardiography in mitral stenotics within the present limitation of the x-ray generator was explained.
   Dr Rink commented on the optimum position for anaesthetisation of mitral stenotics undergoing operation.
   Dr Allanby recorded the circulation times of Doris Diggins and a brief discussion followed on the correlation of these circulatory findings and those shown in angiocardiography, especially in the case of Mary Stewart.
6. The provisional date for the next meeting was fixed for 11th October and the meeting was closed at 11.00 pm.

Maurice Campbell 8/XI/48

---

* See Glossary for venesection.
  An operation recorded as mitral dilatation was performed on her by Mr Brock on 16th September 1948. Unlike Bailey and Harken who published when they had their first survivor, stayed his pen until he had done eight operations, two of them at John Hopkins, with six out eight surviving.

The Heart Club

14

(5) D' Zak presented the cardiac catheterisation report on Doris Diggins (mitral stenosis)

The policy of refraining from angiocardiography in mitral stenosis with the present limitation of the X-ray generator was explained.

D' Rink commented on the optimum position for anaesthetisation of mitral stenotics undergoing operation

D' Allanby recorded the circulation times of Doris Diggins + a brief discussion followed on the correlation of these circulatory findings and those shewn in angiocardiography, especially in the case of Mary Stewart.

The provisional date for the next meeting was fixed for 11th October and the meeting was closed at 11·00 pm.

Maurice Campbell

8/XI/48

The second page of the minutes of 13th September 1948 signed by Maurice Campbell at the November meeting. The club had discussed patients with mitral stenosis. Doris Diggins was probably the first that Brock operated on. Dr Rink the anaesthetist was helping plan the operation which was the first undertaken at Guys. It was yet another very late night for the Peacock Club members.

Tom Treasure

Statistical Table of Operations for Chronic Valvular Disease

Case	Author or Operator	Date	Diagnosis	Method or Instrument	Result	
1.	Doyen [1]	1913	Congenital pulmonary stenosis; patent interventricular septum	Tenotome	Died, few hours after operation	
2.	Tuffier [2]	1914	Aortic stenosis	Finger dilatation	Recovery, improved	*alive*
3.	Cutler and Levine: Boston M. & S. J. **188**: 1023, 1923	5/20/23	Mitral stenosis	Tenotome	Died, 4 years and 6 months after operation	*lived 4 years*
4.	Allen and Graham [4]	8/ 7/23	Mitral stenosis	Cardioscope	Operative death	
5.	Cutler, Levine and Beck [5]	10/ 7/23	Mitral stenosis	Tenotome	Died, 10 hours after operation	
6.	Cutler, Levine and Beck [5]	1/12/24	Mitral stenosis	Tenotome	Died, 20 hours after operation	
7.	Cutler, Levine and Beck [5]	2/25/24	Mitral stenosis	Cardiovalvulotome	Died, sixth day after operation	
8.	Cutler, Levine and Beck [5]	6/11/24	Mitral stenosis	Cardiovalvulotome	Died, third day after operation	
9.	Souttar [6]	5/ 6/25	Mitral stenosis and aortic insufficiency	Finger dilatation	Recovery, living and improved	*alive*
10.	Pribram [7]	11/14/25	Mitral stenosis and aortic vegetative endocarditis	Cardiovalvulotome	Died, sixth day after operation	
11.	Cutler and Beck (first report)	12/ 8/26	Mitral stenosis	Cardiovalvulotome	Died, 15 hours after operation	
12.	Cutler and Beck (first report)	4/15/28	Mitral stenosis	Cardiovalvulotome	Died, 3 hours after operation	

Totals: 12 cases
1 aortic stenosis, acquired
1 pulmonary stenosis, congenital
10 mitral stenosis, acquired

2 finger dilatations
4 tenotome attempts
5 cardiovalvulotome attempts
1 cardioscope attempt

Mortality, 83 per cent

The table of all patients who had a published record of an operation for valve stenosis up to 1929 including all 10 patients who had operations for mitral stenosis. The marginal notes are on the page of the bound copy in the library of Royal Society of Medicine. Only Lilian Hine operated on in 1925 by Souttar[36] was alive at the time of the final report by Cutler and Beck in 1929.[39]

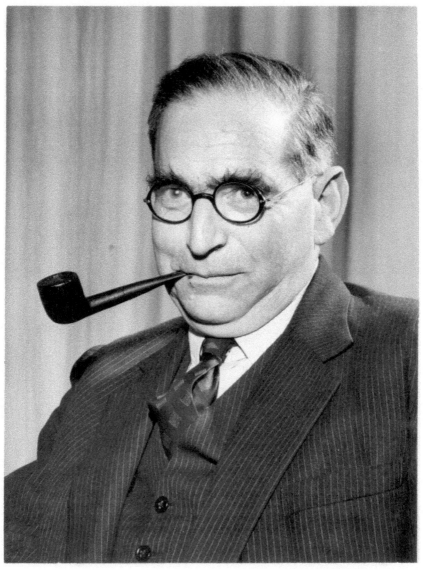

Dr Ernest Herrmann Rink (1903–1959)

November 1948
Minutes of a meeting of the Peacock Club held on Monday 8th November 1948.

There were present:
Dr Campbell, in the chair, Mr Brock, Dr Baker, Dr Rink, Dr Hills, Dr Holling, Dr Zak, Dr Allanby, Mr Channell, Mr Hill and Mr Soothill.

The Minutes of the last meeting were read and approved.

It was agreed that Dr Reynolds, as registrar of the Cardiological Department was ex officio eligible for membership* of the Peacock Club, and should be invited to attend the next meeting.

Dr Campbell then gave a summary of an analysis of 460 cases of congenital heart disease that he had seen since September 1947. Of these 100 were acyanotic and he only proposed to review the 340 who were cyanotic at rest. Of these it would appear that half survived to the age of seven, one in five to the age of 14 and only one in ten to the age of 21 years. During the period under review 43 patients died; but several of these were only seen first in their terminal illness and therefore represented such a highly selected series that analysis was invalid. In the series of cases that had been followed for some time, 25 had died whilst under observation, 24 being cyanotic at rest and one acyanotic. Of these seven died in infancy and had all been given a bad prognosis in view of their history of repeated attacks of unconsciousness, and it seemed that operation below the age of three was of doubtful value. Six died from infection in childhood (three being meningitis deaths) and the remainder died cardiac deaths.

Only 28 autopsies giving the anatomical lesion were obtained in the 41 deaths. 14 were typical Fallots tetralogies, 4 Fallots with an additional deformity, 4 valvular pulmonary stenoses with no ventricular septal defect, and 6 mixed malformations.

---

* See membership in the Glossary of terms.
Ventricular septal defect in the Glossary.

The Heart Club

Dr Allanby then shewed the specimens of the complete cases of Bradshaw, Stewart, Krystodoulu and Coates. In particular the pulmonary valves of Bradshaw and Stewart were compared and the thickened areas and vegetations noted.* In both hearts there were small nodules on the tricuspid valves and in view of the fact that both had been catheterised in life, the possibility of cause and effect was raised. Whilst it was agreed that the catheterisers were supported by experimental evidence that trauma to the valves did not occur in animal experimental catheterisations, there was room for a very healthy scepticism of the innocuousness of the manoeuvre in that no adequate quantity of human material had been sufficiently critically examined. It was decided that all autopsy material should be scrutinised in future in an effort to elucidate the problem.

The question of the aetiology of the lipoid pneumonia in the specimen of Krystodoulu was discussed, and it was agreed that whilst it was not apparent that the cause of death was related to the diodone, no satisfying cause of death was evident, and cyanosis might well have been a deciding factor.

In the specimen of Coates the chief discussion centred around the subvalvular and the valvular elements of the stenosis and the extent to which the valvular narrowing was secondary to the subvalvular reduction of blood flow and the bearing that this had on the planning of direct operative attack on the stenosis.

Dr Hills reported his follow-up of Kuriakou who, since his operation, had returned to Cyprus, and noted the value of this case as propaganda much welcomed by the British school of surgery in Cyprus.§

The date of the next meeting was provisionally fixed for 6th December 1948 and it was agreed that the complete case of Valerie Farmer and Mrs Shakespeare should be discussed fully with all relevant angiocardiograms, catheterisation reports, electro-cardiograms, operative findings and pathological specimens. The remainder of the time was to be spent on

---

* See vegetation in the Glossary.
See lipoid in the Glossary.
See Glossary for diodone.
§ See under Cyprus in the Glossary.

Tom Treasure

the discussion of new angiocardiograms and their correlation with other investigations.

It was suggested by Dr Allanby and generally approved by the meeting that Professor Willis be invited to give us his views on the subject of the development of the pulmonary valve at the meeting in the New Year.

There being no further business, the meeting was concluded at 10.45 pm.

Maurice Campbell
Dec 9th 1948

The Heart Club

December 1948
Minutes of a meeting of the Peacock Club held on Thursday December 9th 1948 at 8.15 pm

There were present, Dr Campbell in the chair, Mr Brock, Dr Baker, Dr Hills, Dr Rink, Dr Kauntze, Dr Suzman, Dr Holling, Dr Allanby, Dr Zak, Mr Channel, Mr Hill and Mr Soothill and Dr Reynolds.

1. The angiocardiogram of Valerie Farmer was shewn and discussed and the possibility of better delineation of the ductus* by retrograde aortography mooted. The angiocardiograms of Janine Lonsdale were then shown to demonstrate the absence of severe pulmonary stenosis as demonstrated by the opacification of the pulmonary vessels themselves and the recirculation in the aorta. It was agreed that an effort should be made further to elucidate the problem by cardiac catheterisation.
   The films of Hilary Druce, Ann Adams and Anita Lang were also viewed before the meeting retired to the Wardens House.
2. The minutes of the previous meeting were read and approved and it was observed that a case that had come to autopsy since the last meeting showed small tricuspid nodules without having undergone cardiac catheterisation in life.
3. The term subvalvular was discussed and after various anatomical excursions it was agreed that the term should be abandoned in preference to infundibular when describing the site of pulmonary stenosis.
4. Dr Campbell announced that he had approached Professor Willis on the subject of the next meeting and it was agreed that this meeting should take place on Monday 19th January 1949, and the venue, at Prof. Willis request would be in the department of Anatomy.
5. Mr Brock raised the question of a cardiac stimulator and artificial pacemaker and stressed the urgency of having this apparatus available in the theatre. He also asked that a further attempt should be made to solve the problems of obtaining satisfactory electrocardiograms during operations. It was agreed that this matter should be tackled and preliminary tests made to estimate the extent and source of interference.

---

* See ductus in the Glossary.
See pacemaker in the Glossary.
See electrocardiogram in the Glossary.

The question of the value of phonocardiograms* in diagnosis and in the keeping of comparable pre- and post-operative records was also raised; but decisions on this subject were indefinite and further information of the details and capabilities of the machine were awaited.

6. Dr Allanby then showed the specimens of the following complete cases: Valerie Farmer as an example of a case of complete pulmonary atresia, with the pulmonary blood supply derived entirely from a patent ductus arteriosus,

A case aged 4 months with pulmonary atresia, an interventricular defect and an overriding aorta.

Mrs Shakespeare as a case of partial transposition.

7. The meeting was concluded at 10.30 pm

Maurice Campbell 10/1/49

---

* See phonocardiogram in the Glossary.
 See transposition in the Glossary.

The Heart Club

January 1949
Minutes of a meeting of the Peacock Club held on Monday 10th January 1949

There were present:

Dr Campbell in the chair, Professor Willis, Dr Foxon, Mr Brock, Mr Whitehead, [sic]* Dr Holling, Dr Allanby, Dr Zak, Dr Brinton, Dr Reynolds, Dr Suzman, Dr Baker, Dr Rink, Dr Channel, Mr Hill and Mr Soothill.

1. The minutes of the previous meeting were read and signed.
2. Professor Willis then gave an account of the development of the heart. He described first the formation and fusion of the heart tubes and their elongation relative to the pericardium causing the bending and folding, and the breakdown of the dorsal mesocardium to form the transverse sinus. He passed rapidly over to venous absorption which formed the definitive venae cavae and atria and proceeded to the septation mechanism. He described the development of the ventral and dorsal endocardial cushions and how the pars membranacea septi was formed from them. The interventricular septum which precedes the interatrial was shewn by models to form from the primitive septum, the endocardial cushions and the right and left spiral bulbar ridges. From this, the formation of the mitral tricuspid orifices and the spiral aortopulmonary septum followed.
   The subdivision of the atria by the septum primum & secundum & the consequent ostia were described and the whole of the process demonstrated by a series of sections of an embryo heart.
   The valves were described as arising from bulbar endocardial proliferations (four in number) in the case of the aorta and pulmonary arteries and from the muscle tissue in the case of the atrioventricular valves. The rotation and subdivision mechanism giving the classical form and position of the aortic and pulmonary valves was demonstrated.
   Professor Willis favoured the view that pulmonary and aortic abnormalities were due to anomalous absorption of the bulbar ridges, and the pulmonary vascular stenosis was a fusion rather than a developmental anomaly & should be contrasted with an infundibular stenosis.

---

* I believe this to be Mr Whythead. See Biographical Notes List 1

Tom Treasure

3. Dr Foxon then gave an account of his work on Ranine circulation. He said that he found it difficult to accept the current views on the function of the spiral septum in the frogs heart and demonstrated angiocardiograms obtained by injecting Thorotrast into a pulmonary vein. These failed to shew that the spiral septum produced any selective distribution of blood, dye* passing equally into cephalic, general systemic and pulmonary arterial systems.

   He noted that in the frog, the atrial septum developed before the ventricular and that though the investigation had little direct bearing on the problem of congenital heart disease in the human, he did feel that considerable caution should be exercised when postulating direction of flow of blood in hearts with incomplete septa.

4. After a brief discussion the meeting closed at 10.15 pm

March 14th 1949 Maurice Campbell.

---

* See dye in the Glossary.

The Heart Club

20

Minutes of a meeting of the Peacock Club held on Monday 18th January 1949

There were present:

Dr Campbell in the chair, Professor Willis, Dr Toxon, Mr Brock, Mr Whitehead, Dr Holling, Dr Allanby, Dr Zak, Dr Brunton, Dr Reynolds, Dr Suzman, Dr Baker, Dr Rink, Dr Channel, Mr Hill & Mr Soothill.

① The minutes of the previous meeting were read & signed

② Professor Willis then gave an account of the development of the heart.

He described first the formation & fusion of the heart tubes & their elongation relative to the pericardium causing the S bending & folding, and the breakdown of the dorsal mesocardium to form the transverse sinus. He passed rapidly over the venous "absorption" which formed the definitive venae cavae and atria & proceeded to the septation mechanism. He described the development of the ventral & dorsal endocardial cushions, & how the pars membranacea septi was formed from

January 1949. Rupert Willis was an authority on comparative anatomy and embryology.[271]

from them. The interventricular septum which precedes the interatrial was shewn by models to form from the primitive septum, the endocardial cushions & the right & left spiral bulbar ridges. From this, the formation of the mitral & tricuspid orifices and the spiral aorto pulmonary septum followed.

The subdivision of the atria by the septa primum & secundum & the consequent ostia were described & the whole processes demonstrated by a series of sections of an embryo heart.

The valves were described as arising from bulbar endocardial proliferations (four in number) in the case of the aorta & pulmonary arteries & from the muscle tissue in the case of the atrio ventricular valves. The rotation & subdivision mechanism giving the classical form & position of the aortic & pulmonary valves was demonstrated.

Professor Willis favoured the view that pulmonary & aortic abnormalities were due to anomalous absorption of the bulbar ridges, and the pulmonary valvular stenosis was a fusion rather than a developmental anomaly & should be contrasted

January 1949. As Brock began his direct operations on pulmonary stenosis he had to work blind within the right ventricle. The Peacock Club went to the basic scientists to study the anatomy.

The Heart Club

with an infundibular stenosis.

3) Dr. Foxon then gave an account of his work on Ranine circulation. He said that he found it difficult to accept the current views on the function of the spiral septum in the frog's heart and demonstrated angiocardiograms obtained by injecting Thorotrast into a pulmonary vein. These failed to shew that the spiral septum produced any selective distribution of blood, dye passing equally into cephalic, general systemic & pulmonary arterial systems.

He noted that in the frog, the atrial septum developed before the ventricular & that though the investigation had little direct bearing on the problem of congenital heart disease in the human, he did feel that considerable caution should be exercised when postulating direction of flow of blood in hearts with incomplete septa

4) After a brief discussion the meeting closed at 10·15.

March 16th 1949. Maurice Campbell

January 1949. The biologist Dr Foxon warned against postulating the direction of blood flow based on extrapolation from structure. He had performed cine angiocardiography on frogs hearts and was ahead of clinical use.[216;217;218;219;230]

Tom Treasure

March 1949
Minutes of a meeting of the Peacock Club held on the 14th March at 8.15 pm

There were present:
Dr Campbell in the chair, Mr Brock, Dr Kauntze, Dr Channell, Dr Baker, Dr Hills, Dr Holling, Dr Brinton, Dr Suzman, Dr Zak, Dr Reynolds, Mr Hill and Mr Hume.

1. The minutes of the previous meeting were read and signed.
2. Dr Channell then demonstrated the specimens of the following complete cases:
   a. Leslie Hamilton who died of bilateral popliteal* emboli. This was demonstrated as a case of the Ebstein malformation. A critical examination of the catheterisation report was made by Dr Zak and of the angiocardiogram by Dr Hills. These examinations appeared to shew a functional pulmonary stenosis.
   b. Elizabeth Metcalfe who shewed an aortic incompetence and a thrombus in the right pulmonary artery. The angiocardiogram was compared with the specimen.
   c. Ronald Pearcey as a case of pure pulmonary stenosis. The shunt demonstrated on the angiocardiogram had occurred through the patent foremen ovale, there being no interventricular defect. Mr Brock stressed the lesson learnt from the recovery of the failing right ventricle after the burden had been relieved by valvulotomy.§
3. A discussion was opened by Dr Zak on the site of the anastomoses of the natural collateral circulation in these cases of congenital heart disease and the bearing that this had on the saturation values found at catheterisation.
4. Dr Campbell raised the question of the preparation of specimens in the future, in view of impending changes in staff.

---

* See popliteal in the Glossary.
  See Ebstein anomaly in the Glossary.
  See aortic incompetence in the Glossary.
§ See valvulotomy in the Glossary.

The Heart Club

5. The date of the next meeting was provisionally fixed for 4th April, when Drs Holling and Zak promised to report their experience with the pulmonary ventilation tests.
6. The meeting was closed at 10.20 pm

Maurice Campbell 4/4/49

Tom Treasure

April 1949

Minutes of a meeting held on Monday 4th April 1949, at 8.15 pm in the library of the Department of Pathology.

There were present:

Dr Campbell in the chair, Mr Brock, Mr OConnell, Dr Baker, Dr Kauntze, Dr Holling, Dr Zak, Dr Suzman, Dr Brinton, Dr Stevens, Dr Hills, Dr Channell, Mr Hill, Mr McLaren and Mr Hume.

1. The minutes of the previous meeting were read and signed.
2. Dr Holling then opened a discussion of the Bing test.[*] He considered it first of all as a simple exercise test, using it as an index of capability more reliable than a patients uncorroborated statement, and more simple and reliable in these cases than the more complicated ergometer tests. He discussed the questions of height, rate and the measurement of exercise in patients of differing size and weight and noted that complicating factors were introduced when considering periods of rest during the test, the possibility of overwork, the effect of training and practice, deformities of the patient such as a hemiplegia, and the extent of cooperation of the patient. Of Bings test itself, with a 9 step climbed 30 times in one minute, Dr Holling felt inclined to offer the following criticisms: Too brisk for the patient trained to take life at a slow pace, too hard for the cardiac patient, heating caused (a) discomfort and the duration of one minute was too short.

    Considered as a ventilation test, the question of accuracy of measurement had to be examined. Bing, using a Douglas bag and gas analysis apparatus estimated an error of 15% and using a spirometer as 25%, though this latter method saved a great deal of time in estimation.

    A demonstration of the application of a graded exercise test was then given using Dr Brinton as the subject, and Dr Holling presented the following conclusions as the result of his limited experiences:

    The one case of Eisenmengers complex[§] did not stand out from the cases of Fallots Tetralogy, and whereas it was easy to distinguish the

---

[*] See Bing test in the Glossary and Bing in Biographical Notes List 2.

See the Glossary for Douglas bag.

Spirometer in the Glossary.

§ See Eisenmenger in the Glossary.

normal from the abnormal heart, it was uncertain when assessing the degrees of abnormality. The early fall in ventilation efficiency seen in heart disease was only shewn in a graded exercise test and not in the single constant exercise of the Bing Test. One serious criticism of the test as at present used was that varying results were obtained from the same patient at different times. In short, it appeared to be of doubtful diagnostic value, but was more useful as an exercise test.

Dr Zak then considered the test from a critical theoretical view point. Quoting from A.V. Hills work he emphasized Dr Hollings criticism that the test was too short and that a steady state could not be reached, even in these cases of heart disease, in one minute.

He considered first of all the minute volume and quoted references to shew that variations in this figure might change as much as 40% from day to day. Emotional factors were of importance and the difficulties with the face piece in the uninitiated, the vagaries of respiratory reflex coordination and the effects of carbon dioxide retention all caused the minute volume to vary out of proportion with the oxygen consumption. These factors were even more important when considering cardiac cases than with normal individuals, for Cournand and Richards[*] found that in normal patients the volume was 3.20 litres/sq.m./min, with a S.D. of 0.65 at rest, 9.70 L/sq.m/min. with S.D. 1.81 at slight exercise and that Knipping and Moncrief had shewn that in dyspnoeic and potentially dyspnoeic patients under exercise increased their minute volume out of proportion using the inefficient rapid shallow respiration.

Considering the oxygen consumption, Cournand and Richards had shewn that even in a control group of normals, a much greater standard deviation of the mean was found on exercise. Another factor was that it would appear that in the case of pulmonary stenosis where the pulmonary flow was limited on exercise, the pulmonary arterial blood was less saturated than normal and yet he believed that the pulmonary vein blood was still fully saturated. This state of affairs was maintained

---

* Referring to work published in 1946 from NYU, Columbia and Bellevue where Zak later worked.[56]

 Possibly referring to work published in 1932 from Eppendorf Hospital, Hamburg.[57] Dr Zak had come from Vienna sometime soon after 1938. Knipping published again in 1950[58] and the MRC team may well have been aware of their work through conferences.

in part by the increased gas pressure gradient in the lungs and by slow pulmonary circulation and would lead to an increased absorption of oxygen compared with the actual pulmonary flow, which might be smaller than indicated by the fall in oxygen consumption.

Dr Zak therefore pleaded for a test to measure the excess oxygen uptake (at the end of a standard test) over the oxygen uptake per unit surface area at rest. The work should be proportional to the body surface rather than to the weight alone. If these values were compared with those of normal individuals it should be possible to draw valid conclusions on the magnitude of the pulmonary flow and the extent of the stenosis. He felt that Bings test was of value in assessing ventilation efficiency in patients with normal pulmonary flow, but of limited value in patients with normal ventilation. There are, in cardiac and dyspnoeic patients, factors other than pulmonary stenosis which produce a lowering of the ventilation index at rest and an even greater lowering with exercise.

Dr Campbell, in reply to Dr Holling said that he felt there was no risk in over exercising the patient in the tests described: but as it was noted that it was the policy to spare these patients all exercise leading to increased cyanosis as it had been assumed that this increased the operative risk. It was apparent that too large a topic had been opened for discussion at this time in the evening, and the meeting was concluded at 10.20 pm after deciding that the next meeting should be held on 2nd May.

May 2nd 1949 Maurice Campbell

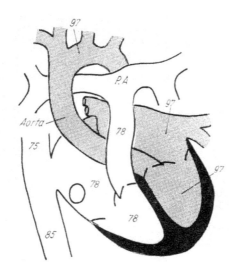

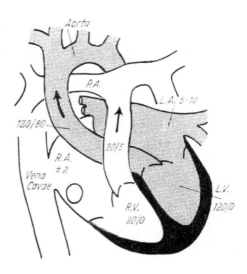

These drawings and normal values are from A Surgeons Guide to Cardiac Diagnosis by Donald Ross published in 1962.[326] The Club members, notably Dr Holling and Dr Zak, were involved in the beginnings of cardiac catheterisation.[231] By withdrawing blood samples for the measurement of the oxygen saturation they could detect and quantify mixing of red and blue blood due to septal defects within the heart. They could also measure pressures in the heart and adjacent blood vessels. In my time as a student and resident at Guys, charts such as these were in use to record the findings of cardiac catheterisation in our patients. They would have been devised during the life of the club.

May 1949
Minutes of a meeting of the Peacock Club held in the Department of Radiology on Monday 2nd May 1949 at 8.15 pm

There were present:
Dr Campbell in the chair, Dr Gardner, Mr Brock, Dr Hills, Dr Holling, Dr Reynolds, Dr Zak, Dr Rink, Dr Baker, Dr Suzman, Mr Whitehead, [sic] Mr Hill and Mr McLaren

1. Dr Gardner demonstrated some full-sized angiocardiograms made at the Royal Free Hospital and a discussion was held on the diagnosis of the cardiac conditions represented.
2. The minutes of the previous meeting were read and approved.
    Dr Campbell then gave a review of the first 50 angiocardiograms performed at Guys, and demonstrated selected cases of films with Dr Hills. Of the 50, thirty-two were considered to be typical Fallot types of malformation. The overriding aorta was in all cases easily shewn at 2 to 3 secs, but the estimation of the degree of pulmonary stenosis proved much more difficult and in those cases checked by catheterisation there was no high correlation with the radiographic opinion and the conclusion drawn was that an apparently good pulmonary blood flow on angiocardiography in no way contraindicated operation.
    There were three cases of Fallot plus a patent ductus or (functional) truncus arteriosus, Susan Atkinson, Derek Scott and Margaret Stone, and these films were demonstrated.
    The next group was one of tricuspid atresia as diagnosed by apparent Fallots with electrocardiographic left axis deviation and in this were the cases of Holliday and Chapman.
    A single case of Pulmonary valvular stenosis with patent foramen ovale was* represented by Doris Savigar, in whom the inter atrial shunt had been demonstrated.
    The Eisenmenger Syndrome appeared to be rare and the only angiocardiogram of this type was that of Olive Davis. In this case of radiological estimation of the excess pulmonary blood flow was hindered by the peculiar appearance of the lung fields on the plain films.
    Lastly the films of Jannaway were shewn as a problem in diagnosis and

---

* See foramen ovale in the Glossary.

The Heart Club

as an example of the complexity of the problem of the interpretation of the results of this radiological investigation.

3. The date of the next meeting was provisionally fixed for Monday 13th June 1949 when Mr Brock hoped to be able to give an account of the result of his work on the development of the infundibular region.

4. The meeting then adjourned to the Wardens House to discuss informally some of the more recent problems.

Maurice Campbell June 13th 1949

Tom Treasure

June 1949
Minutes of a meeting of the Peacock Club held on Monday 13th June 1949 at 8.15 pm.

There were present:
Dr Campbell in the chair, Mr Brock, Dr Rink, Dr Suzman, Dr Reynolds, Dr Brinton, Dr Holling, Mr Channell, Mr Whitehead, [sic] Mr Hill and Mr McLaren.

The minutes of the previous meeting were read and approved.

Dr Campbell then asked Mr Brock to give an account of his investigations into the development of the infundibulum* of the heart.

This, Mr Brock described as a chamber formed in abnormal development of the pulmonary canal, and noted that in Keiths series of 300 cases of congenital abnormality of the heart, most of the abnormalities occurred in this region.

The most important aspect was the muscular arrangement and clues were to be found both in the study of the normal embryology and in the comparative anatomy.

Firstly he briefly recalled the normal development of the heart that had been presented to the club in the meeting of January 1949, stressing the five sections of the primitive heart tube, sinus venosus, atrium, ventricle, bulbus and truncus.

From the comparative aspect, photographs of specimens of skate and ray hearts were shown to demonstrate the bulbus and the musculature and in passing Mr Brock quoted Keith in stating that the human pulmonary valve was incompetent under pressure and that its competence depended on the muscle of the bulbus. The next specimen was of a reptilian heart shewing the aortae arising from the posterior bulbar compartment and compared with the human heart in which the portion of the bulbus nipped off by the

---

* See infundibulum in the Glossary.

interventricular septum formed the aorta, its maldevelopment played a part in congenital aortic stenosis.*

In the absorption of the bulbus the muscle normally grows into the wall of the bulbus as far as the valves.

Next Mr Brock referred to the development of the ventricle, mentioning particularly the sphincteric action of the crista supraventricularis, which is formed as a muscle mass on the medial wall of the infundibular chamber – muscle which has invaded the bulbar ridges as they grow into the lumen of the canal.

In the question of the Tetralogy of Fallot, this muscle mass runs down to the moderator band, and when the question of relieving the stenosis surgically was considered the position of the atrio-ventricular bundle here was of importance. It had frequently been argued as to whether the septal defect or the stenosis was the more important factor in producing the disability in these cases. Hunter described one case of congenital morbus cordis in which he considered the stenosis to be primary factor; Meckell regarded the septal defect as primary; but Peacock supports Hunter in believing that the stenosis causes more blood to be forced into the aorta, pushing the aorta further to the right and maintain the septal defect and causing the dilation of the aorta.

Dissections of sheep hearts were then shewn to demonstrate the outer circular and inner longitudinal arrangement of the infundibular muscle.

Mr Brock then gave an account of the types of infundibular stenosis encountered:

1. An immediate subvalvular stenosis with a poorly developed pulmonary artery. In this case the position of the moderator band indicates that only part of the infundibulum fails to develop.
2. A fibrous ring with overlying muscle.

---

* See aortic stenosis in the Glossary.

Tom Treasure

3. A definite bulbar chamber above the stenosis, with a varying quantity of muscle growing into the wall of the chamber. The crista is fixed and therefore the inlet to the chamber swings until in the extreme type.
4. There is a large chamber above the stricture with an oblique septum.
5. Variations on the extent of the muscle in the outer wall and the site of stenosis on the crista.

When discussing the mechanism of varying shunt, Keith was quoted in believing that the infundibular muscle had a different function from that of the ventricle and that by its varying tonus, it varied the pulmonary blood supply. It was suggested that periods of increased tonicity in the infundibular muscle might correspond with the attacks of cyanosis experience by these children with morbus cruleus.[*]

As a final observation. Mr Brock mentioned that in cases of transportation there is an anti-clockwise rotation so that the new aorta is in the position of the reptilian right aorta. The relative position of the crista supraventricularis supports this observation and it is to be noticed that whereas aortic stenosis is rare in the normally positioned aorta, it is relatively common in the transposed aorta.

The specimen from which the slides had been made were then demonstrated.

The meeting was closed with an appreciation, given by Dr Campbell, of all the work involved in the preparation of this stimulating report by Mr Brock.

Sept 19th 1949 Maurice Campbell

---

[*] See Glossary for morbus cruleus.

The Heart Club

September 1949
Minutes of a meeting held on 19th Sept 1949

Those were present:
Dr Campbell in the chair, Mr Brock, Dr Holling, Dr Reynolds, Dr Zak, Dr Brinton, Dr Suzman, Dr Hills, Mr Hill, Dr Jordan [sic].*

1. Recent angiocardiograms were discussed in Dr Hills office.
2. The meeting then adjourned to the anatomy department to examine the dissected specimen of Sheila Rowe, John Nudd, Margaret Rose and Katherine Lowery.
3. It was decided not to hold a meeting in August.
4. The meeting was adjourned at 10.00 pm.

Maurice Campbell
November 8th 1949

---

* Appeared for some meetings as Jordan but I have seen his name in the operating book, committee minutes when his attachment was extended, and on several published papers and Michael Jordaan seems the only likely candidate.[236;237;238]
An occasion when the date of the signature and next meeting date do not align.

Tom Treasure

November 1949
Minutes of a meeting held on Monday 7.11.49.

There were present
Dr Campbell in the chair, Dr Hills, Dr Brinton, Dr Holling, Dr Zak, Dr Reynolds, Mr Hill, Dr Soothill, Dr Jordaan.

1. The angiocardiograms of Howard, Waring and Williams were discussed.
2. The minutes of the previous meetings were read and approved.
3. The next meeting was provisionally fixed for Monday 12th December and it was decided to invite members of the Heart Hospital Staff.
4. Specimens of the following complete cases were shewn:
   Priam, as a case of situs inversus with partial transposition.
   A case of Fallots Tetralogy with endocarditis and vegetations causing a machinery murmur.
   The specimen of Ivy Viccars with the complete anastomosis which had not functioned owing to kinking over the aorta.*
   The specimen of Beaumont with congenital aortic aneurism.
5. The meeting closed at 10.00 pm.

---

* This was a recognised mode of technical failure with a Blalock shunt.[28]
  Undated in the original

The Heart Club

December 1949
Minutes of a meeting held on Monday 12th December 1949 at 9.00 pm.

There were present:
Dr Campbell in the chair, Mr Brock, Dr Kauntze, Dr Deuchar, Dr Holling, Dr Zak, Dr Allanby, Dr Brinton, Mr Channell, Dr Reynolds, Dr Rink, Mr Whytehead, Dr Jordan [sic],* Mr Hill, Mr Brown, and by invitation, Dr. Paul Wood, Dr. Darke, Dr.Somerville, Dr. Magidson, Dr. Woods, Dr McGregor, Dr Whitaker, Dr Schrire, Dr Abrahams & Dr Lowe.

Dr Campbell called on Mr Hill to give a short paper on angiocardiograms.

Firstly the apparatus and methods were described, and the limitations of the present speed shewn with slower full size plates for comparison. The venous routes used were demonstrated by films. A series of films was then shewn to illustrate some of the conditions other than cyanotic congenital heart disease which had been investigated by this method.

Next the value of P.A. films were discussed, particularly from the point of view of the surgeon and several films were demonstrated which had influenced the side and route of approach, and the type of operation to be performed, and the common fallacies in interpretation noted.

From the point of view of direct cardiac surgery§ it was felt that the detail of intracardiac anatomy was at present inadequate on the small films and that in selected cases there was a great part to be played by the full-size film, even though the series was less complete.

---

* As previously noted, this must be Michael Jordaan whose name is in medical committee minutes and he later published on Club topics after returning to South Africa. See Biographical Notes List 1.

These last six were guests from the Heart Hospital as planned in the previous meeting.

The original typed minute is unclear as to whether Dr or Mr was intended but as Dr (Tom) Hills, the radiologist, is not listed and the Hill is quite distinct I believe it was the surgical senior registrar Ian Hill making the presentation. In support of that conclusion is a later paper with Ian Hill as sole author in which it is clear that he was the operator in many of the angiocardiograms done around this time.[51]

§ See the Glossary for direct cardiac operations.

Tom Treasure

Finally several angiocardiograms were put up for discussion of the diagnosis and interpretation.

Dr Brinton then demonstrated several specimens, including two of which angiocardiograms were available for comparison. The value of in vivo observations was stressed by Mr Brock, who noted the fallacies that might arise in making unqualified observations of the fixed, hardened specimens of an organ that was in life a functioning muscle mass.

The meeting ended after a general discussion at 11.00 pm.

6/2/50 Maurice Campbell

The Heart Club

34

```
Minutes of a meeting held on Monday 12th December 1949
at 9.0 p.m.

There were present :---
Dr Campbell in the chair, Mr. Brock,Dr. Kauntze,Dr.Deughr
Dr. Holling,Dr. Zak,Dr. Allanby,Dr. Brinton, Mr. Channel,
Dr. Reynolds, Dr. Rink, Mr.Whytehead, Dr. Jordan, Mr. Hill,
Mr. Brown, and by invitation, Dr. Paul Wood, Dr. Darke,
Dr. Somerville, Dr. Magidson, Dr. Woods, Dr. McGregor,
Dr. Whitaker, Dr. Schrire, Dr. Abrahams & Dr. Lowe.

Dr. Campbell called on Dr. Hill to give a short paper on
angiocardiograms.
     Firstly the apparatus and methods were described,
and the limitations of the present speed shewn with slower
full size plates for comparison.  The venous routes
used were demonstrated by films.  A series of films
was then shewn to illustrate some of the conditions other
than cyanotic congenital heart disease which had been
investigated by this method.
     Next the value of P.A. films was discussed, pariculaly
from the point of view of the surgeon and several films
were demonstrated which had influenced the side and route
of approach, and the type of operation to be performed,
and the common falacies in interpretation noted.
     From the point of view of direct cardiac surgery it
was felt that the d tail of intracardiac anatomy was at
present inadequate on the small films andthat in selacted
cases there was a great part to be played by the full size
film, even though the series was less complete.
     Finally several angiocardiograms were put up for dis-
cussion of the diagnosis and interpretation
     Dr. Brinton then demostrated several specimens,
including two of which angiocardiograms were available
for comparison.  The value of invivo observations was s
stressed by Mr. Brock, who noted the fallacies that might
arise in making unqualified observations of the fixed,
hardened specimens of an organ that was in life a functionin
muscle mass.
     The meeting ended after a general discussion at 11 p,m;
```

6/2/50   *Maurice Campbell*

The group by invitation led by Dr Paul Wood at the December 1949 meeting were the clinical and research staff from the National Heart Hospital. It is an interesting but an inevitable fact that a specialist heart hospital could not pioneer heart surgery because it had as yet no surgeons or surgical facilities. Guys and the Brompton Hospital (where Brock also worked) had thoracic surgeons who were ready, willing and to varying degrees, able to turn their hand to cardiac surgery. Paul Wood was later a co-author on the first 100 mitral valvotomy paper.[118]

Tom Treasure

February 1950

Minutes of a meeting of the Peacock Club held on Monday 6.2.50 at 8.15 pm

There were present:
Dr Campbell in the chair, Mr Brock, Dr Baker, Dr Kauntze, Dr Rink, Dr Hills, Dr Holling, Dr Brinton, Dr Reynolds, Dr Zak, Dr Deuchar, Mr Brown, Mr Channell, Mr Whytehead, Dr Jordaan, Mr Bates & Mr Hill.

Dr Campbell asked Mr Brock to give a brief account of some of the matters of interest in his American visit.

Mr Brock first passed briefly over the angiocardiograms at the Johns Hopkins--- A-P & Lateral views with a Fairchild camera* and always under local anaesthetic, the cardiac catheterisation, especially Bings work and the use of the oximeter.

He then came to the question of the general acceptance of the Blalock type of anastomosis for the cases of congenital cyanotic heart disease, and mentioned the question of refrigeration and the type of case upon which Potts was operating.

In passing he appraised the system of the Forum and gave his impressions of the type and standard of the experimental and clinical work that he had seen at the various centres that he had visited. In particular he singled out the work of Gross in Boston, and the use of arterial grafts and Blalocks work on the cases of transposition and Becks work in the revascularisation of the heart.

Finally, Mr Brock gave a brief account of his own work at the Johns Hopkins Hospital including the series of seven pulmonary valvulotomies with one death and two mitral valvulotomies. He felt that the operation of pulmonary valvulotomy in the cases of pure valvular stenosis had been accepted by the Johns Hopkins.

---

* See Fairchild camera in the Glossary.
 Probably referring to total body cooling. See hypothermia in the Glossary and the illustration of a patient undergoing surface cooling.
 See the Glossary with respect to the use of valvotomy and valvulotomy.

The Heart Club

In connexion with the work on Mitral stenosis he particularly mentioned the work of Bailey, Glover and ONeill in Philadelphia* and the attitude of many American physicians to the direct and indirect surgical methods of treating this disability.

In the discussion which followed, Dr Campbell first spoke, mentioning particularly the nursing standard in America, and the whole question of the use and abuse of the recovery room was discussed generally, and Dr Baker commented on his experience in his recent visit.

Finally, Dr Brinton shewed the specimens of the complete cases of Peter Wilson, Christine Hayward and Raymond Smith.

It was agreed that the next meeting should be held on 6th March 1950, and Dr Campbell agreed to give an account of the follow-up of the direct cardiac operations.

The meeting concluded at 10.30 pm

R.C. Brock

---

* This is Charles Bailey and his colleagues who had their first survivor at their fifth attempt.[48] See the opening chapter on Guys 1945-8 for a note on the early operations for mitral stenosis.
  Undated in the original. Probably 6th March when Brock chaired the meeting.

> Minutes of a meeting of the Peacock Club held on
> Monday 6.2.50 at 8.15.p.m.
>
> There were present Dr. Campbell in the chair, Mr. Brock,
> Dr. Baker, Dr. Kauntze,Dr. Rink,Dr. Hills,Dr. Holling,
> Dr. Brinton, Dr. Reynolds,Dr. Zak,Dr. Deuchar,Mr. Brown,
> Mr,Channell, Mr. Whytehead,Dr. Jordaan, Mr. Bates & Mr.Hill
>
> Dr. Campbell aske Mr. Brock to give a brief account   t
> of some of the matters of interest in his American visit.
>   Mr. Brock first passed briefly over the angiocardio-
> grams at the Johns Hopkins--- A-P & Lateral views with
> a Fairchild camera and always under local anaesthetic,
> the cardiac catheterisation, especially Bing's work and
> the use of the oximeter.
>   He then came to the question of the general
> acceptance of the Blalock type of anastomosis for the
> cases of congenital cyanotic heart disease, and mentioned
> the question of refrigeration andthe type of case upon whic
> Potts was operating.
>   In passing he appraised the system of the"Forum"
> and gave his impressions of the type and standard of the
> experimental and clinical work that he had seen at the
> various centres that he had visited.   In particular
> he singled out the work of Gross in Bostong and the
> use of arterial grafts and Blalock's work on the cases
> of transposition and Beck's work in the revascularisation
> of the heart .
>   Finally Mr. Brock gave a brief account of his own work
> at the Johns Hopkins Hospital including the series of
> seven pulmonary valvulatomies with one death and two
> mitral valvulatomies.   He felt that the operation of
> pulmonary valvulatomy in the cases of pure valvular
> stenosis had been accepted by the John's Hopkins.
>   In connexion with the work on Mitral stenosis he
> particularly mentioned the work of Bailey, Glover &
> O'Neill in Philadelphia and the attitude of many
> American physicians to the direct and indirect surgical
> methods of treating this disability.

The February 1950 meeting included an important mention of Brocks operations at Johns Hopkins on both mitral and pulmonary stenosis. They later decided to change their terminology from valvulotomy to valvotomy.[118] This copy of the original typed minutes reveals some uncertainty about the spelling, at least on the part of the typist.

The Heart Club

BRITISH MEDICAL JOURNAL

LONDON SATURDAY JUNE 3 1950

VALVULOTOMY FOR MITRAL STENOSIS
REPORT OF SIX SUCCESSFUL CASES
BY

CHARLES BAKER, O.B.E., M.D., F.R.C.P.

R. C. BROCK, M.S., F.R.C.S., F.A.C.S.(Hon.)

AND

MAURICE CAMPBELL, O.B.E., M.D., F.R.C.P.

(From the Cardiac Department and the Thoracic Surgical Unit, Guy's Hospital)

It is now a quarter of a century since a number of attempts were made to relieve mitral stenosis by operation. The most sustained efforts to solve this problem by direct attack on the valves were made by Cutler and his associates (Cutler and Beck, 1929). Their first patient survived four years and was thought to have been improved ; six others died soon after operation, as also did single cases reported by Allen and Graham (1922) and by Pribram (1926). Souttar (1925) alone has published a further success in an important paper from this country.

These early efforts were succeeded by a long period of inaction, and many thought that direct surgery of the valves of the heart was too dangerous to be practicable. The need for reconsidering this has become increasingly clear during recent years, because great advances in thoracic surgery and anaesthesia and in the aftercare of the patient have entirely changed the prospects of success. That successful operations for the direct relief of valvular stenosis are possible was shown in the case of the pulmonary valve (Brock, 1948) ; and that successful resection of infundibular stenosis was also possible was shown in the following year (Brock, 1949). We have performed in all over 45 direct operations on the heart for the relief of these types of stenosis.

While this work was being developed during the last four years our attention was also directed towards the relief of mitral stenosis by direct operation on the mitral valve. We are now able to report eight such cases, six of which are successful. These clinical results show that operation is not only possible but holds out hope of relief for a number of sufferers from this crippling condition.

That we have tried to select our cases with proper caution, recognizing the inherent dangers and difficulties, is shown by the fact that out of the many patients seen during this time only a few were specifically considered for surgery. In addition, the first patient selected was observed for more than a year before operation was finally decided on and performed in September, 1948.

At the same time that we were engaged with this problem several teams in America were similarly occupied. With some workers the approach has been indirect : Bland and Sweet (1949) have devised and practised a venous-shunt operation in which an anastomosis is made between the azygos vein and a branch of the inferior pulmonary vein,

with the intention of relieving the high pressure in the pulmonary circulation. D'Allaines and his colleagues (1949) have used a similar operation in Paris. Harken, Ellis, Ware, and Norman (1948, 1950) have used both direct and indirect septal defect in two patients, and operation upon the mitral valve itself in two patients with one death. Smithy (1949), before his untimely death, operated directly upon the mitral valve in seven patients with two deaths. Murray (1949), of Toronto, mentions two patients in whom he has resected one cusp of a stenosed mitral valve and inserted a section of cephalic vein to function as a new valve.

The largest number of operations upon the valvular stenosis itself have been done in Philadelphia by Bailey, Glover, and O'Neill, who have developed a technique similar to the one we have used. Up to February, 1949 (Bailey, 1949), they had operated upon 10 patients with three successes, but in a later report (Bailey, Glover, and O'Neill, 1950) they mention 22 patients with 11 survivals ; when we visited their clinic they had already passed this figure with more successes and a lower mortality.

Selection of Cases for Operation

This is difficult, as substantial reasons on which to base our opinions can come only as more patients are operated on. From many patients with mitral stenosis only a few have been selected as suitable for valvulotomy ; in this we have been conservative and have waited until it is clear that the patient is deteriorating and that prognosis without operation is bad. The decision to operate earlier, before changes are so far advanced, and a widening of the field of indications, will depend on the results of surgery, and so far they are encouraging. The possibility of surgery should, we think, be remembered so that the right type of case may be helped at the right time.

The therapeutic problem presented by mitral stenosis involves many more features than the narrowed valvular orifice. Treatment must be considered in relation to the natural history of the disease ; the liability of rheumatic carditis to recur or to smoulder ; the involvement of the other valves ; the usual coexistence of some slight or gross degree of incompetence of the valve ; calcification of the valve ; the development of pulmonary hypertension with secondary changes in the pulmonary arteries and the lungs ; the onset of auricular fibrillation ; and, above all,

4665

The first publication on surgery for mitral stenosis from the Guys group including those done by Brock at Johns Hopkins. [63]

Tuesday, June 6, 1950

Hospital Fire—No Neglect

THE fire which resulted in the death of a doctor and a nurse at Brompton Hospital, Fulham Road, London, on May 27, started in an X-ray-film storage room, said Dr. Frank Kingman, of the Joint Fire Research Organisation, at yesterday's resumed inquest. The cause of ignition could not be found out.

The Hammersmith coroner, Mr. H. Neville Stafford, said: "That, to my mind, is the most disturbing element of this inquiry."

He recorded verdicts of "Accidental death" on Dr. Gerald Channell, aged 39, of Knebworth, Herts, and Nurse Evelyn Mary Roberts, aged 30, of Grassdale, Liverpool. There was no evidence of neglect or carelessness by the hospital authorities.

The February 1950 meeting was the last recorded attendance of Gerald Channell. He went to the Brompton for surgical training but was killed in a fire started in an x-ray film store. He had worked in anatomy and was acknowledged posthumously for his contribution to dissections of necropsy specimens. [185]

The Heart Club

March 1950
Minutes of a Meeting of the Peacock Club held on Monday 6th March 1950 at 8.15 pm.

There were present:
Mr Brock in the chair,[*] Dr Campbell, Dr Baker, Dr Brinton, Dr Reynolds, Mr Whytehead, Dr Jordaan, Mr Brown, Mr Barrett, Mr Cleland & Mr Hill.

Mr Brock called upon Dr Campbell to give an account of the follow-up of the cases of direct cardiac operation.

Dr Campbell said that he was only including the cases operated upon up to the time that Mr Brock left for America – 11 valvulotomies and 11 infundibular punch resections.

Of the valvulotomies, 6 were pure valvular stenoses, 4 were in extremis and there were 5 deaths, though the survivor was one of the most remarkable successes. The remaining 5 were Tetralogies and in these cases there was only one death. In the survivors there was one excellent result, (arterial O_2 91% satn.) one good result and two fair results.

To this series should be added the 8 cases in America with only one death.[§]

In the 11 cases of infundibular resection there were three deaths, all over the age of 19 years. Of the 8 survivors, 7 shewed a very great improvement.[¶]

---

[*] It was unusual for Brock to chair but this may have been because Dr Campbell was presenting on a subject close to Brock or perhaps the visit of some senior London surgeons had some bearing on it.
 Brown, Barrett and Cleland were thoracic surgeons in other hospitals in London (see biographies) possibly invited because Brock was reporting on his exchange visit to Johns Hopkins.
 The original has valvulatomies which I regard as typists error which is likely given the change in nomenclature.
[§] Publishing in 1950 Blalock wrote The operation is that which has been described by Mr. Brock of Guys Hospital, London, and in fact he performed the operation on seven of the patients described in this report while he was serving as an Exchange Professor in The Johns Hopkins Medical School and Hospital. Slight variations which we have made in Mr. Brocks technic are without significance.[178]
[¶] Brock and Campbell were preparing this work for a report in the *BHJ*.[59]

Tom Treasure

The cardiac enlargement that follows these operations is roughly the same as that which follows the Blalock type of procedure and he felt that this was rather an increase in the chamber size than an increase in the size of the wall.

The E.C.G. changes with the direct operations--- ST bowing with TI inversion---- go after six weeks except in the chest leads and the R.V.P.* persists.

Mr Brock then commented on the survey and noted that three of the deaths in the valvulotomy series occurred before the actual cardiac operation had been performed and that perhaps a truer picture of the risk in suitable cases was presented by the complete series of 20 cases performed at the Johns Hopkins by Blalock and himself with only one death.

In the infundibular series, two of the deaths were in cases diagnosed at operation as valvular stenosis and found at autopsy to have high infundibular stenosis with granulations and progressive fibrosis making them unsuitable for the direct attack.

Finally he reiterated the value of procaine, both intravenously and topically in these operations and said that increased safety might lie in the approach to the stenosis through the infundibular chamber, where this was anatomically feasible, in that it would reduce the stimulation of the sensitive ventricle which might respond to the incision in its wall with uncontrollable irregularity.

Dr Reynolds confirmed that the E.C.G. tracings taken at operation definitely shewed less irritability since the adequate use of procaine.

In the subsequent discussion of heart specimens Dr Brinton and Mr Barrett spoke.

The meeting was concluded at 10.15 pm.

R.C. Brock 17.4.50

---

* Right ventricular predominance.
  See procaine in the Glossary.

The Heart Club

April 1950
Minutes of a meeting of the Peacock Club held at 8.15 pm on Monday 17.4.50.

There were present:
Mr Brock in the chair, Dr Baker, Dr Suzman, Dr Holling, Dr Zak, Dr Trounce, Dr Brinton, Dr Deucher, Mr Whytehead, Mr Jordaan and Mr Hill.

After the minutes of the previous two meetings had been read and approved, Mr Brock asked Mr Brinton to read his paper on the investigation of blood levels before and after operations for congenital heart disease.*

Dr Brinton stated that he had analysed the figures from 138 cases in which the average preoperative values for Haemoglobin was 21.7G % R.B.C 8.07M, Hct. 69.4%, M.C.Hb. concentration 31, and M.C.V. 86 c. He noted that the Hb content was roughly proportional to the R.B.C. until 29G% and that after 6 million the M.C.H. fell.

The preoperative oxygen saturation shewed no correlation on a scatter diagram with the Haemoglobin value, but in view of the fact that decreasing oxygen tension affected haemoglobin formation before cell poiesis, preoperative iron might raise the M.C.H.C.

He then discussed the significance of scatter diagrams plotting the following factors: Mean cell volume and R.B. count, Haemoglobin M.C.H.C and M.C.H. and R.B.C., mean corpuscular haemoglobin and mean cell volume, mean cell volume and Haemoglobin; M.C.H.C. & M.C.H. c HG, Haemoglobin and packed cell volume.

Next the findings in 60 operated cases were recorded and discussed. The results were divided into five categories; 5 outstanding, in which the blood picture change corresponded with the clinical improvement; (all these had normal preoperative M.C.H.C.); 10 very good, in which 7 cases the clinical and haematological findings agreed, 22 good, 22 fair and 1 slight.

---

* This works was published in Guys Hospital Reports during 1951[60-62]
Hand corrected and unclear in the original.

Tom Treasure

In the postoperative haemoglobin fall, 59% were stable in three weeks. Those with normochromic M.C.H.C. (32.5) all fell at first and then returned to normal, whilst those hypochromic all rose without a fall. The M.C.V. in all cases tended to return to normal.

In the discussion that followed, Mr Brock thanked Dr Brinton for the work involved in such detailed and careful presentation of the subject.

Dr Hollings shewed a scatter diagram of preoperative Hb. Concentration plotted against effective pulmonary blood flow. If the E.P.B.F. logarithmic values were plotted against Hb. Values, nearly all the points fell within the limits of 20% above or below the curve.

The meeting concluded with an examination of recent complete specimens.

Sept 25th 1950 Maurice Campbell

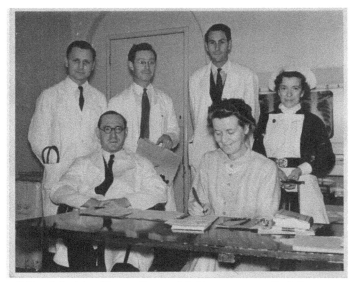

Russell Brock in his office at Guys with his secretary Chris Jones next to him. When Brock was widowed, she became Lady Brock. Immediately behind Brock is Ian Hill and the nurse is Sister Fallwasser. She lived in her rooms next to the ward and nursed many patients through difficult recoveries. The other two men will be members of the surgical team and probably Peacock Club attendees but they have not been identified.

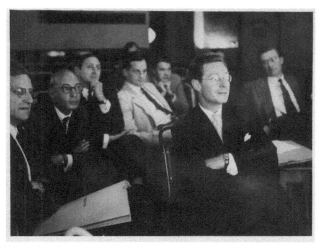

Ian Hill in the foreground of a group in a conference. It might well have been a Peacock Club meeting. The man on the extreme left has x-ray packets on his lap and might be Dr Tom Hills but that has not been confirmed.

Tom Treasure

September 1950
Minutes of a meeting of the Peacock Club held at 8.15 pm on Monday 25th
September 1950

There were present:
Dr Campbell in the chair; Dr Brinton, Mr Brock, Dr Deuchar, Mr Hill,
Dr Hills, Dr Holling Dr Reynolds, Mr Scott, Dr Suzman, Dr Trounce,
Mr Whytehead, Dr Zak, and by invitation Mr Barrett, Mr Cleland,
Dr Cooley, Dr Raymond Daley, and Dr ONeill.

1. The minutes of the previous meeting were read and approved.
2. It was decided to include the subject of mitral stenosis and of acquired
   heart disease generally in the club activities.[*]
3. Mr Barrett asked a question on the subject of nature of the Peacock Club
   and visitors and Dr Campbell in replying indicated the essentially Guys
   nature of the club.
4. Dr Hills raised the problem of an X ray theatre and the type of work
   to be done there was discussed and a sub-committee of Mr Brock, Dr
   Campbell and Dr Deuchar was suggested further to look into the matter.
5. Recent complete specimens from Guys and the Brompton Hospital
   were shewn illustrating both unoperated and operated congenital and acquired cardiac condition(s) in this discussion. Dr ONeill of
   Philadelphia spoke on his experience of the surgery of mitral stenosis
   and shewed several slides.

The meeting was concluded at 10.15 pm.

Nov 27th 1950 Maurice Campbell

---

[*] Baker, Brock and Campbell had published their results for surgery of mitral stenosis in the BMJ in June 1950.[63]
 The team in Philadelphia had also published on the surgery of mitral stenosis.[48;64-66]

The Heart Club

> Minutes of a meeting of the Peacock Club held at 8.15pm on Monday 25th Sept 1950
>
> There were present:—
> D Campbell in the chair; D Brinton, M Brock D Donohoe, M Hill, D Hills, D Holling, D Reyne, M Scott, D Suzman, D Trounce M Whytehead; by invitation M Barrett, M Cleland D Cooley, D Raymond Daley & D O'Neill.
>
> (1) The minutes of the previous meeting were read & approved
> (2) It was decided to include the subject of mitral stenosis & of acquired heart disease generally in the club's activities
> (3) M Barrett asked a question on the subject of nature of the Peacock Club & Dr Campbell in replying indicated the essentially "guys" nature of the club.
> (4) D Hills raised the problem of an X ray theatre & the type of work to be done there was discussed and a sub-committee

The attendance on 25th September 1950 included several visiting surgeons. Denton Cooley who assisted Blalock at Johns Hopkins was working at the Brompton and was an early adopter of mitral valvotomy.[199] Mr Barrett was thoracic surgeon at St Thomas Hospital and Mr Cleland at the Hammersmith Hospital. Evidently Norman Pasty Barrett was not welcomed as a member by Dr Campbell.

The second page of the Minutes for the meeting in September 1950, signed by Maurice Campbell on 27th November 1950. Dr ONeill was a colleague of Charles Bailey, the first to have success with surgery for mitral stenosis in the 1940s era.[65;66]

The Heart Club

November 1950
Minutes of a meeting of the Peacock Club held at 8.15 pm on Monday 27.11.50

There were present:
Dr Campbell in the chair, Dr Baker, Mr Brock, Mr Hill, Dr Holling, Dr Reynolds, Mr Scott, Dr Suzman, Dr Trounce, Mr Whytehead, Dr Zak, and by invitation Mr Judson Chesterman.

The minutes of the previous meeting were read and signed.
1. Arising: Dr Campbell stated that the business of the subcommittee mention in para 4 of the minutes of the previous meeting had been satisfactorily completed without the meeting of the committee.
2. The secretary, being no longer on the Guys strength expressed his wish to resign office.* Dr Holling was nominated as the next secretary, to take over in 1951.
3. It was decided to hold the next meeting on 15th Jan 1951 and that the subject of Preoperative Assessment of Mitral Stenosis should be discussed.
4. Dr Reynolds agreed to give a short paper on electrocardiographic changes during angiocardiography at a future date.
5. Dr Baker then opened the discussion on arrhythmias following mitral valvulotomy. Reviewing 23 cases (20 at Guys), 8 were fibrillating before operation and 5 died, 3 of embolism: 15 had preoperative normal rhythm, 3 died but 5 fibrillated later (3 on 3rd day and 2 on 14th day). This raised the question of digitalisation before operation in cases likely to fibrillate and whether any warning of fibrillation could be obtained from E.C.G. at operation.
   In the matter of treatment Dr Baker favoured digitalis control rather than quinidine§ reversion, where fibrillation may later recur. He felt that the digitalised fibrillating patient ran less risk of tachycardiac complication.
   Mr Brock mentioned five Brompton cases and raised the question of the use of Cortisone.

---

* This was Ian Hill.
That is treatment with digitalis. See the Glossary for digitalis.
See fibrillation in the Glossary.
§ See quinidine in the Glossary.

Dr Suzman mentioned the possibility of treating fibrillation with effusion by hyaluronidase to the pericardium.

The matter of pericardial anaesthetisation in preventing neurogenic fibrillation was discussed and the fact that temporary postoperative fibrillation might well be post thoracotomy instead of post cardiotomy. Dr Campbell therefore favoured the use of quinidine in the postoperative case as opposed to the mitral stenotic fibrillator. The question of postoperative murmur change was briefly mentioned, several specimens shewn and the meeting concluded at 10.30 pm.

January 15th 1951
Maurice Campbell

The Heart Club

January 1951

Minutes of a meeting of the Peacock Club held at 8.15 pm on Monday January 15th 1951.

There were present:

Dr Campbell in the chair, Dr Baker, Mr Brock, Dr Deuchar, Mr Hill, Dr Holling, Dr Reynolds, Dr Suzman, Dr Trounce, Mr Vant Hoff, Dr Venner, Dr Zak and by invitation Dr Cosh, and Dr Knebel.

Dr Holling opened a discussion on the investigation of patients with mitral stenosis. He considered a scheme suggested by Dr Baker to grade the patients on clinical grounds. The difficulty was to find objective tests whose results would run parallel to these. Exercise tests were difficult to evaluate.

The pulmonary congestion which is supposed to be caused by mitral stenosis could be measured in a number of ways. The actual volume of blood in the lesser circulation could be measured but the results showed that this was not increased in mitral stenosis.

Maximum breathing capacity seemed to be a good method of measuring the loss of elasticity of the lungs which was diminished in mitral stenosis. The decrease in alveolar air space is not sufficient to be detectable by measurement of the residual air of the lungs. Vital capacity measurements were being done and might prove valuable. Measurement of the efficiency of the lungs in terms of volume of oxygen removed from each litre of air breathed had not proved to be satisfactory. Slight diminution of the oxygen saturation of the arterial blood could be shown in cases of mitral stenosis.

Cardiac catheterisation gave a means of measuring the restriction of the circulation caused by the stenosis. In order to be able to compare the results of one case with those of another it was necessary that the patients should be in a basal state at the time of catheterisation, but this was very difficult to achieve. In any case the clinical disability of the patient and the reduction in cardiac output did not appear to run parallel, nor did the elevation take into account the rise in pulmonary artery pressure and the rise in cardiac output might prove to be a useful way of assessing the fitness of the patient.

A tracing of pulmonary venous pressure was shown and its characteristics explained, this measurement seems to be an important one in mitral stenosis since it is thought to be near that of the left atrium. A formula for calculation of the area of the mitral valve was given.

Dr Campbell agreed how important it was to recognise the limitations of laboratory tests. He asked whether it had been noticed that cases of mitral stenosis had rapid shallow respiration in distinction to cases of aortic disease. In congenital heart disease pulmonary hypertension and disability did not go together.

Dr Baker stressed the importance of coming to a clear decision about ones clinical assessment of the disability of a patient in some cases who had emphasised their symptoms the objective tests had been useful. He pointed out that we were dealing here not only with pure mitral stenosis but with some patients who had other lesions in addition. The scheme put forward was really quite a simple one

Dr Suzman asked whether there was any relationship between the size of the left atrium and the severity of the case, Mr Brock thought not.

Mr Hill reminded the meeting that the only check on the physiological investigations which we had was a really careful investigation of the case clinically.

Dr Zak thought that the combined measurement of cardiac output and pulmonary artery pressure during exercise appeared to be useful. Measurements of lung ventilation required time and patience and the results could not always be relied on. He did not think that it was necessary to worry about getting an accurate figure for the cardiac output it was sufficient to show that it was reduced.

The measurement of pulmonary venous pressure was not a straightforward measure because it was difficult to be sure how securely the catheter was blocking the pulmonary vessel. It was also important to take into account the position of the catheter in the chest, for this might make a difference of as much as 10 mm Hg to the recorded pressure.

The Heart Club

Dr Cosh suggested that the nitrous oxide method of measuring cardiac output might prove less upsetting to the patient and had the advantage that it could be frequently repeated.

Dr Deuchar thought that the opening speaker had adequately shown how little use physiological tests were. Unfortunately little reliance can be placed on the statement of a patient or his relative about his condition and he frequently found this when dealing with cases of congenital heart disease.

Dr Venner gave the figures which showed that a case of mitral stenosis might continue to improve for some months after operation.

The meeting concluded at 10.20 pm.

February 12th 1951 Maurice Campbell

Tom Treasure

February 1951

Minutes of a meeting of the Peacock Club held in the wardens House, Monday, February 12th, 1951, at 8.15 p.m.

There were present:

Mr Brock (in the chair), Dr Baker, Dr Brinton, Dr Campbell, Dr Deuchar, Mr Hill, Dr Hills, Dr Holling, Dr Reynolds, Dr Susman [sic], Dr Trounce, Dr Venner, Dr Verel, Mr Whytehead, Dr Zak, and by invitation Dr Dubost of LHopital Broussais, Paris, and Dr Knebel.*

The minutes of the previous meeting were read and approved.

The date of the next meeting was provisionally arranged for March 5th, the subjects for discussion to be Selective Angiocardiography opened by Dr Hills, and The Heart Catheterisation of Congenital Heart Disease by Dr Deuchar.

Dr Campbell then described his study of the relationship between the radiological appearances and the blood pressure and blood flow in the pulmonary vessels. He paid tribute to Helen Taussigs pioneer work in the subject, and mentioned his own nomenclature of oligaemic and pleonaemic lung field – descriptive terms which had not given satisfaction in all quarters. Until the introduction of the cardiac catheter it was difficult to confirm or deny theories about the radiological appearances. The hilar shadows appear to be caused by arteries and not by veins; perhaps this was because the four pulmonary veins each carry only half the amount of blood which the two pulmonary arteries carry. Pezzi, an Italian, introduced the graphic term hilar dance[§] which was a term rather easier to use than to define.[¶] Such increased pulsation might occur in atrial septal defect, patent ductus arteriosus, ventricular septal defect, transposition of the great vessels, and Eisenmengers syndrome.

---

* Dr Knebel remains unidentified. In the original of Wurtzberg had been typed and very deliberately crossed out.

  See Glossary for oligaemic.

  Pleonaemic is the converse – radiologically demonstrated excessive blood flow to the lungs.

§ Hilar dance is in the Glossary.

¶ Campbells detailed account of this was published in the *BHJ* that year.[67]

The Heart Club

The relationship between the size of the pulmonary arteries and the degree of pulsation in them together with the pulmonary blood flow and the pulmonary arterial pressure was shown in the following table.

49.

	Usual range.			Pulsation.			
	Pulm. flow l./sq.m./min.	Pressure, mm. Hg	Size of Rt. P.A.	Rt. P.A.	Mid-zone.	Periphery.	Hilar dance.
P.D.A.	6-23	Normal to 50/30	++	2	1	-	-
A.S.D.	9-20	Normal to 45/20	++ (+)	3	3	2	Yes
V.S.D.	9-23	40/15 to 120/60	++	3	3	2	Yes
Transposition	5-9	About 90/50	+++	3	2	2	Yes
Eisenmenger	2-3	95/55 to 155/95	+++	3	2	-	-
Mitral stenosis.	2-4	40/25 to 120/60	++ (+)	1	-	-	-

Pulmonary regurgitation was often present with V.S.D. and Eisenmenger's complex but not so often in other groups.

The arterial O2 saturation was normal in P.D.A. and A.S.D., between 89 and 98% in V.S.D. and reduced in Eisenmenger and Transposition.

Though all these cases showed enlarged pulmonary arteries marked pulsation was seen only in the cases of A.S.D., V.S.D., transposition, and Eisenmenger's syndrome. The pulsation in mitral stenosis was not markedly increased.

Thus it would seem that increased pulsation is more to be ascribed to increased pulmonary flow than to increased pulmonary artery pressure. There were, however, two patients who had greatly increased pulsation but had high pulmonary arterial pressure and low pulmonary artery flows. It was also difficult to explain the increased

Pulmonary regurgitation was often present with V.S.D. and Eisenmengers complex but not so often in other groups.

The arterial 0_2 saturation was normal in P.D.A. and A.S.D., between 89 and 98% in V.S.D. and reduced in Eisenmenger and transposition.

Though all these cases showed enlarged pulmonary arteries marked pulsation was seen only in the cases of A.S.D., V.S.D., transposition, and Eisenmengers syndrome. The pulsation in mitral stenosis was not markedly increased.

Thus it would seem that increased pulsation is more to be ascribed to increased pulmonary flow than to increased pulmonary artery pressure. There were, however, two patients who had greatly increased pulsation but had high pulmonary arterial pressure and low pulmonary artery flows. It was also difficult to explain the increased pulsation in Eisenmengers Complex, unless this condition represented the late stage of a ventricular septal defect. Possibly as Dr Reynolds had suggested, the pulsation was less in P.D.A. than in A.S.D. and V.S.D., because the latter conditions would be expected to give more abrupt change in pressure.

Dr Campbell had found the diameter of the right pulmonary artery increased in Transposition and Eisenmengers Complex, less increased in A.S.D. and only slightly increased in P.D.A. and V.S.D.

Dexter, though dealing with older patients, had produced similar figures to those of the Guys cases.

pulsation in Eisenmenger's Complex, unless this condition represented the late stage of a ventricular septal defect. Possibly as Dr. Reynolds had suggested, the pulsation was less in P.D.A. than in A.S.D. and V.S.D., because the latter conditions would be expected to give more abrupt changes in pressure.

Dr. Campbell had found the diameter of the right pulmonary artery increased in Transposition and Eisenmenger's Complex, less increased in A.S.D. and only slightly increased in P.D.A. and V.S.D.

Dexter, though dealing with older patients, had produced similar figures to those of the Guy's cases.

RELATIONSHIP OF SIZE AND PULSATION TO FLOWS & PRESSURES
FROM DEXTER'S FIGURES.

		Size.	Pulsation.	Flow (average)	Pressure. (average)
	Increased flows without increased pressure.				
1.	P.D.A.	1.0	0.6	4.7	28/11
2.	A.S.D.	1.95	1.3	10.3	28/11
	Increased flow and pressures.				
3.	P.D.A.	1.75	0.4	12.5	53/33
4.	A.S.D.	2.7	1.4	12.5	65/30
	Increased pressure without increased flow.				
5.	Eis.	2.25	0.7	2.9	115/60
6.	M.S.	2.0	0.1	3.1	78/40

He thought on the basis of these figures that the effects of increased flow or increased pressure were indistinguishable.

He thought on the basis of these figures that the effects of increased flow or increased pressure were indistinguishable.

Dr Campbell then showed X-Rays of various conditions. In A.S.D. pulsation could be seen beyond the engorged vessels seen in a film. The large nodular looking arteries seen in cases with greatly increased blood flow were very different from the finer mottling of the lungs seen in mitral stenosis. In mitral stenosis there was often an opaque line stretching into the right upper lobe; perhaps this was an engorged vein.

Mr Brock thanked Dr Campbell for his lucid and scholarly communication. The reason why pulmonary veins cannot be seen is because they have short stems and branch quickly so that they are hidden behind the heart. It is seldom that anomalies in their anatomy are encountered in routine chest surgery. The term mid zone could not be used in the sense Dr Campbell suggested because it had been already used to indicate the portion between the 2nd and 4th ribs; perhaps intermediate zone would suit Dr Campbells purpose. The structure Dr Campbell had called R.P.A was perhaps more exactly called right lower lobe artery.*

Mr Hill described how angiography showed the pulmonary veins hidden behind the heart.

In P.D.A. Dr Deuchar had found that the pressure tracings confirmed the suggestion that pulmonary artery pulsation is not marked.

Dr Suzman reminded the meeting that the extent of normal pulsation must be taken into account. In a large artery this might look abnormal. A good working rule to follow is that if increased pulsation is not immediately seen it is probably not present.

Mr Brock asked what were the appearances in cor pulmonale.

---

* This and the comments above about pulmonary veins was anatomical point scoring as thoracic surgeons will recognise.
See cor pulmonale in the Glossary.

The Heart Club

Dr Hills said that pulsation might be more difficult to see in denser lung fields. Perhaps the electro kymograph would be of value in measuring pulsation. It would also be interesting to dissect out and X-Ray against different densities a pulmonary artery and vein.

In Dr Bakers experience pulmonary artery pulsation was even less in mitral stenosis than Dr Campbell had suggested and the changes in the lung fields may be due to haemosiderosis. When A.S.D. was present the pulsation was unmistakable. Had sufficient attention been given to the effects of nervousness.

Drs Campbell and Hill agreed that hilar dance was not seen in normals no matter how increased the pulmonary flow. This was rather against Dr Campbells thesis. The pulsation in nervous subjects does not spread into the lung fields.

Dr Dubost suggested that lateral views might show up the pulmonary veins, and that the engorged veins in mitral stenosis might obscure the pulsation of the arteries.

The meeting closed at 10.30 pm.

March 5th 1951
Maurice Campbell

Tom Treasure

March 1951

A meeting of the Peacock Club was held in the library of the Pathological Department on Monday March 5th 1951 at 8.15pm

There were present Dr Campbell (in the chair), Dr Baker, Mr Brock, Dr Carnegie, Dr Deuchar, Dr Graham, Mr Hills, Dr Holling, Dr Rink, Dr Suzman, Dr Venner, Mr Whytehead, Dr Zak, and by invitation Dr Allanby and Dr Knebel.

Dr Hills said that the Fairchild Camera capable of taking 2 full sized chest X-Rays per second was now available. This made selective angiocardiograms a possibility. A machine to inject 15cc of solution in one second was also available. Before using these devices for selective angiocardiography it would be as well to consider possible dangers. Does the catheter straighten out under the pressure used, and may the contrast medium be injected into the heart wall? Could observations on animals give a guide to the likelihood of these dangers arising?

Mr Whytehead suggested that the total amount to be injected was 15 to 40ml.

Mr Brock spoke of the possibility of injecting dye so quickly into small chambers that they became ruptured. Frances Gardener had experience of the method and her opinion should be asked. He had seen excellent aortograms done by Dr P Woods team in which 60 ml had been given in 2 seconds. It seemed safer to inject along the lumen of a vessel. Oblique and lateral views would be required.

In a discussion of the value of anaesthesia it seemed likely that anaesthesia might be required to eliminate unpleasant sensations but that it should not be made deep enough to eliminate the cough reflex.

Mr Brock remarked that it was easy to go on finding objections, the thing was to get on with the job.[*]

---

[*] For those who knew him this statement captures the determination of Russell Brock.

The Heart Club

Dr Deuchar then reviewed the results of 187 cardiac catheterisations done from November 1947 when Dr Zak introduced the technique to the hospital till the end of 1950. In the last year twice as many catheterisations had been done as in either of the two previous years. The complications met with were similar to those encountered elsewhere.

In Fallots Tetralogy the aorta was only entered in 2 of 34 patients. If the aorta is entered from the right ventricle the likelihood is that the pulmonary opening is atretic. The right ventricular systolic pressure in Fallots Tetralogy varied from 75 to 132 mmHg. (Though Brian Johnstons was 170 mmHg.)

In most cases of pulmonary stenosis the right ventricular pressure was between 135 and 180 though occasionally it was lower. But it seemed that a high right ventricular pressure was in favour of pulmonary stenosis.

Two cases of infundibular stenosis showed a double rise of pressure in withdrawing the catheter from pulmonary artery to right ventricle. The level of stenosis might be estimated by noticing in the X-Ray at what point the pressure recorded increased, but this was not always exact.

It was difficult to compare diagnoses made by catheterisation with diagnoses made without its aid because after all catheterisation was not a method apart from the other clinical investigations.

Dr Campbell said how valuable Dr Deuchars review had been. Mr Brock urged for more post-operative catheterisations and pointed out that the position of a pulmonary stenosis varied throughout the cardiac cycle. Dr Deuchar produced diagrams to show that however the pulmonary blood flow might vary the systemic blood flow remained within normal limits.

This meeting closed at 11.00 pm.
9/4/51 Maurice Campbell

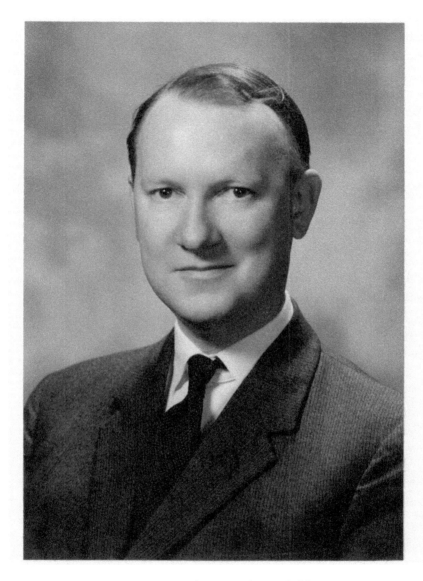

Dennis Deuchar (1924–1977) attended from
December 1949 to March 1953.[27;28;76-8;158;203-208]

The Heart Club

April 1951
A meeting of the Peacock Club was held in the Clinical Amphitheatre on Monday, April 9th, 1951 at 8.15 pm.

There were present Dr Campbell in the chair, Dr Baker, Mr Brock, Dr Deuchar, Dr Graham, Mr Hill, Dr Holling, Dr Reynolds, Dr Suzman, Dr Trounce, Dr Vant Hoff and Dr Venner. Dr Zak, Dr Knebel and Dr Macdonald were present by invitation.

The date of the next meeting was fixed for May 21st, the subject for discussion to be Mitral Stenosis.

Mr Brock then showed films on the surgical treatment of Pulmonary Stenosis.

Dr Trounce showed pathological specimens of Newton, Philpot, Holt and Spiet.

May 21st 1951
Maurice Campbell

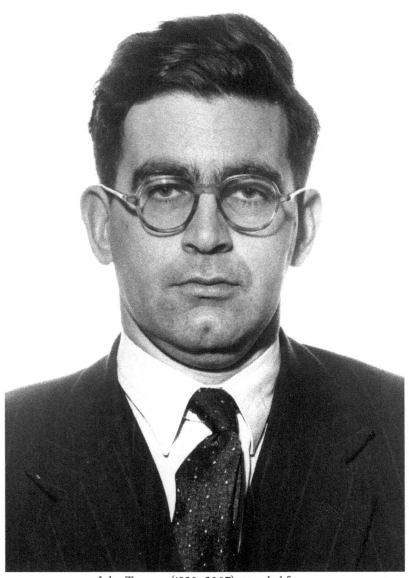

John Trounce (1920–2007) attended from April 1950 to April 1951.[69;116;121;182;264]

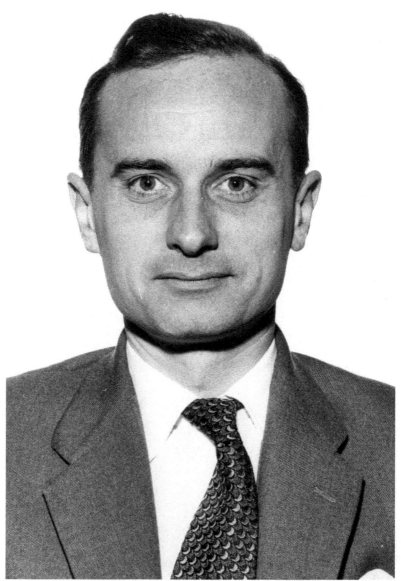

Ian MacDonald (1921–2008) attended once in April 1951.
He taught physiology for many years (1948 to 1977) and was
prominent internationally in nutrition science. He contributed
to a paper on estimating blood oxygen, central to the
investigation of congenital heart disease by catherisation. [235]

Tom Treasure

May 1951

A meeting of the Peacock Club was held in the Wardens House on May 21st 1951 at 8.15pm.

Dr Campbell was in the chair and 16 members attended. The guests were Mr Brown and Dr Somerville.[*]

The date of the next meeting was fixed for July 2nd. The subjects for discussion to be ECGs during angiocardiography (Dr Reynolds). The ECG in mitral stenosis (Dr Trounce) and if time permitted Intra Arterial and Intra Cardiac Pulse tracing. Drs Holling, Venner and Verel.

Dr Baker spoke of the feature of mitral stenosis as seen in over 200 cases attending Guys during the past year. He pointed out that stenosis of the mitral valve was not an isolated anatomical defect in any otherwise healthy patient. Other conditions were also present which might also affect function and prognosis.

The effects of secondary changes in the pulmonary circulation was not known, but in the history of these patients it was surprising how often attacks of so called chronic bronchitis occurred; some of these attacks may be rheumatic manifestations. It is sometimes said that right heart failure may coincide.

Fatigue is a common symptom in mitral stenosis though one which is difficult to assess. The degree of fatigue from which patients had suffered was best seen by comparing a patients energy before and after operation.

Cardiac pain occurred in mitral stenosis more often than was generally realised. In very few of the cases of mitral stenosis was an accompanying neurosis present.

---

[*] Dr Walter Somerville. See Biographical Notes. Also in List 2 Dr Jane Somerville who was only just in medical school but was later (1955/6) Brocks house surgeon.
Reynolds published this work in the *BHJ*.[68]
Trounce published this work in the *BHJ*.[69]

The Heart Club

Clinical Signs
These were not of great help in assessing a case and after a most successful operation there may or may not be a change in the cardiac murmurs.

Dr Baker now found that the size of the left atrium could be assessed from an A.P. film and barium swallow was not required.

Pulsation in the pulmonary vessels was slight and the cause of mottling of the lungs was still not clear.

Diagnosis of mitral incompetence was not greatly assisted by radiology and in a large heart it was difficult to see expansile pulsation of the atrium. Perhaps one could say that mitral regurgitation was minimal if the left atrium was small.

Auricular fibrillation was not a contra indication to operation but was an added risk. Cases with fibrillation were older and had their condition longer than those without. The onset of auricular fibrillation may be associated with an embolus but this does not necessarily mean that emboli will be frequent thereafter. A great difficulty is to decide in which case rheumatic infection is smouldering.

Dr Campbell agreed that neurosis is seldom met with in cases of mitral stenosis, and that fatigue occurs often. The disability caused by mitral stenosis has been more clearly recognised since we have been able to see patients before and after a successful operation. He preferred to keep the term angina for use in coronary disease and in cardiac disease generally to speak of sternal pain on exertion.

Dr Sommerville [sic] mentioned the work of Soulie and Balzac which showed that systolic pulsation of the left atrium was a most fallible sign of mitral stenosis. He thought that objective exercise tests should be done to assess the improvement after operation.

Dr Baker said that patients, to a skilled questioner, gave a consistent account of their physical disability.

Dr Campbell also remarked that most men of experience had discarded exercise tests as a means of assessing disability in heart disease.

Dr Suzman wondered whether small hearts and left atria were associated with pulmonary oedema. Dr Baker said there was no correlation. Dr Venner showed the effect of valvulotomy on pulmonary artery pressure. Cases which clinically were greatly improved had had a high pulmonary artery pressure before operation which had fallen greatly after operation. Two cases were moderately improved they had had only moderately raised pressures which had fallen ... *... clinically and he had shown little change in a high pulmonary artery pressure.

Mr Brock said that the actual size of the mitral orifice was of small prognostic importance, in fact all stenosed mitral valves he had felt, with four exceptions, appeared to be of a standard size. The cusps show different lesions and different parts of the ring may be affected to different degrees. The functional capacity of the heart is also important. Cases should not be turned down because of chronic bronchitis because this may itself be a manifestation of mitral stenosis. Detection of expansile pulsation was an unimpressive method of investigation. Now that valvulotomy had been shown of value in some types of cases it was necessary to operate on many types of cases to determine the full usefulness of the operation. Bronchitis, for example frequently clears up after operation.

In reply to a question of Dr Suzman Dr Baker said that only 5 or 6 of the Guys cases had had bouts of congestive failure Mr Brown said that Dexter had been giving ACTH to cases suspected of having rheumatic infection but he had heard that cortisone may lead to mental disorder. Aschoff nodes were frequently found in the amputated auricles but this seemed to be poor evidence of the presence of active rheumatism.

July 2nd 1951 Maurice Campbell

---

* There is a handwritten addition in the original which runs off the page and is curtailed by cropping of the pages in binding.
See Aschoff nodes in the Glossary.

The Heart Club

July 1951

A meeting of the Peacock Club was held in the Clinical Amphitheatre on July 2nd 1951. There were present 15 members and by invitation Drs McMillan[*] and Matthews of St. Thomas Hospital.

The date of the meeting was fixed for September 10th the subject to be Vascular Pressures at Operation.

Dr McMillan described an apparatus he had devised for studying the action of human aortic and pulmonary valves. The apparatus delivers in a pulsatile stream 3 litres of water a minute through the valvular opening. In the films the opening and closing of normal pulmonary and aortic valves was shown, together with examples of calcified, stenotic, incompetent and bicuspid, aortic valves.

Dr Campbell congratulated Dr McMillan on his films. Mr Brock said how useful this apparatus should be in the study of the action of flap valves over the aortic orifice.

Drs McMillan, Brock and Campbell agreed that it would be difficult to show the action of the mitral valves because in a dead heart the papillary muscles would not act normally. Dr McMillan also pointed out that where a live heart contracts with increased pressure a dead heart would dilate. He was however considering the use of a double systole system for this purpose.

Dr Reynolds then read his paper on electrocardiography during angio-cardiography. The study was started after three patients had died shortly after undergoing angiocardiography.[§] It is difficult to find out what the percentage mortality from angiography is; up to 1950 26 deaths had been reported. Electrocardiographic studies during the procedure have been few.

---

[*] I believe this was Ian McMillan who went on to be consultant surgeon in Southampton. He gained his Fellowship of the Royal College of Surgeons in 1956 and prior to that was titled Dr and after that Mr.

Published in the *BHJ*.[70]

Published in the *BHJ*.[68]

[§] The Club were very aware of the risks catheterisation particularly in cyanotic patients and included this in their publications.[71;72]

A Swedish paper on selective angiocardiography reports curves indicating coronary insufficiency when the opaque medium is injected into the aorta.

The present study concerns 75 angiocardiograms done in 73 patients. The majority were cyanotic cases.

Changes in the electrocardiograms followed no set pattern. The heart rate was often 150– 190/mm. and on injection fell by 10 to 20 beats/min. Ectopic beats occurred which may have been caused by the anaesthesia, diodone itself did not appear to cause ectopic beats. Diodone prolonged the PR interval and even resulted in some bundle branch block in 11 cases. Procaine is known to depress conduction in the heart and it may be significant that 13 of 19 cases who showed slowed conduction had had procaine.

Some ST deviation either elevation or depression might take place after the injection but this might also occur before the injection.

In the one fatal case of the series, ST depression in 1 and elevation in 3 occurred quickly after injection. Another case showed similar changes but settled down quickly.

More ECG changes occurred in anaesthetised patients but this might have been as much due to the youth of the patients as to the anaesthetic. One of the 73 cases died, three collapsed at varying times after angiocardiograms. One had a distended stomach, another wet lungs.

The changes in ECG seem to precede clinical changes. The collapse may be due to fall in blood pressure, but may be due to a direct effect on the lungs.

Following the use of procaine ECG abnormalities still occurred though no death had occurred since its introduction. Three severe arrhythmias had occurred and perhaps there was a chance of interfering with the heart action by overdose. Whytehead remarked that procaine in doses of 8–10 mgm/mm was said to help to prevent pulmonary oedema.

In selective angiocardiography at least 2 infarcts had occurred as the result of injection of diodone into the lungs. Mr Brock knew of two more.

The Heart Club

Dr Matthews said that at St. Thomas they had successfully used Pentothal and Flaxedil to abolish the cough reflex.

Dr Campbell suggested that cyanotic attacks might be a sign of danger and that serious cerebral complications had resulted from cerebral anoxemia.

Dr Trounce then discussed electrocardiographic change in 75 cases of mitral stenosis, one third of which had been catheterised.[*]

Right axis deviation and auricular fibrillation were common as many previous workers had found. Changes in p waves previously described had been found but in addition he had found 72% of diphasic p waves in the V1 lead whereas of an unselected group of cardiac cases not more than 17% showed such changes. Flat topped p waves occurred in 61% of cases, notched waves in 31%. The PR interval was prolonged in only 4 cases none showed QT changes. R.A.D. occurred in 48% only one case, which was suspected of aortic regurgitation showed left axis deviation. Evidence of R.V. Hypertrophy was shown in 92% of cases by fluoroscopy. There was no good correlation between the appearance of right ventricular preponderance and increased pulmonary artery pressure.

In summary, biphasic p waves in V1 had been found frequently in these cases of mitral stenosis. There was no correlation between ECG changes size of the right ventricle, or pulmonary artery pressure.

Dr Campbell remarked that RAD was a better indication of right ventricular hypertrophy in Congenital Heart disease than X-Ray appearances. In chronic pulmonary disease right ventricular hypertrophy may occur, though the ECG showed no RVP. In mitral stenosis variable results occurred, perhaps this was due to the effect of rheumatic carditis in the heart muscle.

Dr Suzman asked whether there was any relationship between Pulmonary Artery Pressure and T wave changes. Dr Trounce said that possible relationships of that kind were obscured by the effect of digitalis.

---

[*] Published in the *BHJ.* [69]

Tom Treasure

Dr Trounce showed pathological specimens of Brown, Susan, Turner and Nicholas Craig.

The meeting adjourned at about 11.00 pm.

Oct 1st 1951*
Maurice Campbell

---

* Date of signature does not match the date of the next meeting.

The Heart Club

October 1951

The Peacock Club met in the Wardens House shortly after 8.15 pm on October 2nd, 1951. Dr Campbell was in the chair. There were present 18 members and by invitation Dr Daley of St Thomass Hospital, Dr Starkey of New York and Mr Milstein.

The date of the next meeting was fixed for Monday 12th November, the subject to be angiography, and the opening speaker Mr Hill.

Dr Verel reported some results obtained during the operation of mitral valvulotomy using a fine intra-arterial catheter. The blood pressure during an operation showed three phases. A slightly lowered pressure at the beginning, a further fall some little time after the chest had been opened and a marked fall occurring whilst the valvulotomy was actually being done. Towards the end of the operation the blood pressure often tended to rise but seldom to higher levels than it was at the beginning.

The first small fall of blood pressure might well be due to the relaxation caused by the anaesthesia.

The cause of the second fall was obscure. It was not directly due to opening the chest nor to opening the pericardium, or manipulation of the lung, but it may be due to dislocation of the heart. The courses of the blood pressure and the concurrent events occurring during an operation were shown for a number of cases.

A record of the pulse pressures during the actual opening of the stenosed valve was shown. Dr Verel pointed out how characteristic this was and of what short duration it was. The duration of 50 seconds for a valvulotomy was certainly not the shortest time.

Records of systematic blood pressure were taken simultaneously with the pulmonary artery and left atrial pressure, but so far without showing any evidence that the two were related to each other.

Dr Rink said that the anaesthetist found it a great consolation to have the blood pressure measured at levels lower than 60 mm Hg when the knowledge was most valuable. Without this the anaesthetist had the difficult job of judging the condition of his patient from his pulse rate, his looks and his colour. During the early stages of anaesthesia the blood pressure usually fell from about 120 to 90mm. Hg and slowly fell to 75 mm Hg during the early stages of operation. During the operation it was not unusual for the pressure to drop to unrecordable levels. The severest drop occurred when the pericardium was opened and the heart was palpated. This might happen in a case of congenital heart disease during examination of the pulmonary opening and the rise when the pericardium was closed and a subclavian pulmonary anastomosis performed. The disease of the heart was probably an important factor in causing the fall of blood pressure for with a normal heart these manoeuvres can be done without a great fall in blood pressure.

Dr Campbell said that cerebral complications followed the earlier operations with greater frequency than the later. This change was likely to be due to the fact that now the valvulotomy could be carried out quickly and the patient subjected to a low blood pressure for a much shorter time.

Dr Reynolds said that E.C.G. abnormalities did occur but it was difficult to relate them to what was happening on the operation table because the man at the E.C.G. could not see what was happening on the table. He believed that many of the changes arose from direct stimulation of the myocardium.

Mr Hill said that the intravenous drip of procaine might be a factor in causing the drop in blood pressure, also he believed that procaine in the pericardium might be toxic and perhaps propine [sic]* amide was preferable. Opening the pericardium did not cause a fall in blood pressure but pulling on it did. Dr Verel had not mentioned the fall in blood pressure which occurs on recovery from the anaesthetic. Unless prolonged this need not be taken seriously.

Dr Rink pointed out that the intravenous procaine was started only when the patient was on the table and so was unlikely to be the only cause of the fall in blood pressure. He considered that it was the improvement in cardiac action which followed the valvulotomy which enabled the patient to get through the operation. He knew of two patients who had been operated

---

* Maybe procaine was intended.

on and no valvulotomy done; one of them had died. Deterioration of these patients continues from the start of the operation until the valvulotomy is done.

Dr Daley found that in operations in dogs the pericardium could be opened and the heart palpated without any fall in blood pressure but that this invariably occurred when the heart was dislocated. In the post-operative period a massive effusion was connected with a fall in blood pressure.

Dr Starkey said that a rough intubation of the patient might cause a fall in blood pressure, or if the surgeon was impatient and had the patient put into position on the table too quickly. Usually when the lung is retracted the blood pressure falls.

It is necessary to consider the effect of respiratory disturbances on the circulation. If the anaesthetist is not ventilating the lung adequately sufficient oxygen may be supplied but CO_2 may be imperfectly eliminated. After a difficult intubation the oxygen saturation may remain normal but the CO_2 pressure rises and the p H falls to 7; with this there is a fall in blood pressure. Too much compression of the lung allows the blood pressure to fall and therefore the surgeon should allow the anaesthetist to ventilate the lungs adequately. Beechar and Gibbon have studied this and shown that as the CO_2 is blown off the blood pressure rises.

Hill agreed that inefficient ventilation of the lungs might cause a fall of blood pressure.

Dr Holling mentioned the possibility of reflexes from the mediastinum being responsible for the fall in pressure.

Dr Venner first dealt with the necessity for determining the reference level when measuring pressures and using a manometer with saline filled connection to the manometer. Failure to realise the importance of this may easily cause an error of 100% in measuring the atrial pressure. The reference level favoured was at the level of the 4th costal cartilage in the mid line and midway between the front and back of the chest. If the atrial pressures are referred to this point it is found that left atrial pressures measured at operation by either saline or electric manometer agree fairly well.

The characteristics of the normal left atrial pulse were then described and it was shown how variable such a pulse tracing might be. In order to form any idea of what the various waves in the atrial tracing could mean it was necessary to have synchronous E.C.G. but with his apparatus the difficulties of doing this were only just being overcome. Tracings of right and left atrial and pulmonary capillary tracings were shown. Some of the tracings were too much damped because he had tried to keep well clear of the operation field and to use as small a needle as possible.

The characteristic tracing of mitral regurgitation according to Wiggers is the prolongation of the second positive wave into the ventricular diastole. One patient with mitral regurgitation showed this the other did not. Mitral regurgitation does not appear on the pulse tracings taken after valvulotomy. The atrial pressure falls after a valvulotomy and it has been said that this fall is due to a fall in systemic pressure but this is not true. The interpretation of curves unless one can read a simultaneous E.C.G. is almost impossible.

The pulmonary artery pressures taken at operation agree very well with those obtained at catheterisation, except in three cases. In one case a low pulmonary artery pressure was recorded at catheterisation and a high one at operation. It may be possible to account for the difference in this case because between catheterisation and operation he had developed signs of pulmonary oedema. The other case who had a high pressure at operation had had an attack of pulmonary oedema during the induction of anaesthesia. The third patient had a higher pressure at catheterisation but this investigation had caused some agitation to her. After sternotomy the change in pulmonary artery pressure is not remarkable which is in accordance with the fact that the improvement which follows operation is gradual.

The left atrial pressure at operation is often found to be higher than the pulmonary capillary pressure at catheterisation and there is little relationship between the two. This may be reasonable if the summit of the pulse wave in the pulmonary capillaries is higher than the simultaneous pressure in the atrium allowing blood to flow onwards. The discrepancy between the

The Heart Club

two pressures, however, may be an artefact because at operation the chest is open and the anaesthesia is applying positive pressure. This may cause a rise in atrial pressure and another possibility is that the anaesthetic agent may cause abnormal pulmonary dilatation.

Dr Baker said that even with our present methods of investigation we could not prevent a case of mitral regurgitation coming to operation. The pulmonary capillary tracings did not appear to have been of great value in diagnosing mitral regurgitation.

Dr Venner agreed with this statement and mentioned the difficulties of being sure that the catheter was recording what was the pulmonary capillary pressure.

Dr Campbell doubted that we could measure pulmonary capillary pressures for attempts to measure them from the arterial and venous end of the vessels had shown different results.

Mr Hill pointed out that different mitral valves behave differently; in some the valve balloons back into the atrium with ventricular systole and in others remains in its place; this might alter the pattern of atrial pressure records and possibly of pulmonary capillary records. The best result for valvulotomy came from a valve with a soft diaphragm. Perhaps we should with improvement in diagnosis be able to diagnose the type of valve with which the surgeon would have to deal.

Dr Deuchar said that pulmonary capillary tracings were very difficult to interpret and thought that very often they were nothing but records of respiration. In his experience pulmonary artery and venous capillary tracings agreed and the pulmonary venous pressure was only 3 mm. Hg above that of the left atrium. People who hoped to diagnose ballooning of the mitral valves from pulmonary capillary tracings were optimists.

Dr Verel in answer to a question of Dr Deuchar showed how the time lag of the recordings system could be measured by comparing simultaneous E.C.G.s with ventricular tracings.

Dr Starkey said that Dr Cournand also found pulmonary capillary tracings difficult to obtain and to interpret.

Dr Daley thought that pulmonary venous and capillary pressures as at present measured dont correlate. He had 30 tracings of pressure pulses in normal left atria. Those obtained in mitral stenosis differ from these because in the normals the first wave precedes the Q.R.S. complex and in the mitral curves it succeeds it. Cases had come to operation which did not have a systolic murmur nor a paradoxical expansion of the atrium and yet had mitral regurgitation as shown by the atrial pulse curve. He did, however, think that some pulmonary capillary curves might indicate mitral regurgitation. At operation if the atrial pressure dropped 100 mm Hg a good result was likely. He pointed out that the pulmonary artery pressure might be very variable and he had had the experience of watching the right ventricular pressure in a very excitable Irishman who started by having a severe dyspnoea because he thought he had won a sweep. At that time his ventricular pressure was 90/6 and when he fell into a sleep the pressure fell to 32/5. Later his brachial artery had to be punctured and the pressure rose to 65/5. He thought that a useful pre-operative test was to do a Valsalva to see whether the flow can be increased. If it can, then probably a mitral valvulotomy wont help.

He then showed tracings obtained at operation with a Sanborn manometer[*] showing simultaneous left and right atrial pressure with E.C.G.s.

Dr Reynolds showed three pathological specimens.

November 12th 1951 Maurice Campbell

---

* See Glossary for Sanborn.

The Heart Club

November 1951

At a meeting of the Peacock Club in the library of the Pathological Department, on Monday, November 12th, 1951, there were present fifteen members.

The date of the next meeting was fixed for January 14th, 1952, the subject to be The Surgical Anatomy of the Mitral Valve, the opening speaker, Mr Brock.

Mr Hill reviewed 162 angiographies performed at Guys, 146 of which were on cases of congenital cyanotic heart disease.[*]

At the close of this communication Dr Campbell congratulated the speaker on the honesty of his approach to the subject.

Mr Hill showed a P.M. specimen of Ebsteins Disease which had not been recognised as such by the pathologist, and Dr Scott showed a P.M. specimen of mitral stenosis.

January 14th 1952 Maurice Campbell

---

[*] Published in the *British Journal of Surgery*.[51]

Tom Treasure

January 1952

There was a meeting of the Peacock Club in the staff Common Room at 8.15 p.m. on January 14th, 1952. Twenty members were present. Mr Nicks of New Zealand was a guest.

The date of the next meeting was fixed for February 11th, when Dr Deuchar will speak on records taken at operation on cases of congenital heart disease.

Mr Brock spoke on the surgical anatomy of the mitral valve and the change taking place in it when affected by rheumatism. He pointed out that the valve is a complicated neuromuscular mechanism and not simply a fibrous flap. The usual method of demonstrating a stenosed valve does not show what is appreciated at operation. The valve could, however, be dissected in such a way as to make the important points clear and Mr Brock showed such dissections. The main attachments of the papillary muscles is to two points on the valves about 1 cm apart. When the mitral valve is affected by rheumatism the chordae tendinae become bunched and thickened towards the point of main attachment to the valve at which two masses of fibrous tissue are formed which hold the free edges of the valve cusps together. At operation the mitral orifice is almost constantly about 1 cm by 0.5 cm. which would correspond to the papillary muscles. When the adhesion at the point of papillary attachment is cleared the adhesions between the valves laterally and medially may be very light. These findings suggest that the usually accepted theory that rheumatism first attacks the closure line of the valves making them rough and sticky so that they adhere to each other is not the whole story, at least so far as the mitral valves are concerned. It is suggested that the valve cusps are firmly held together at these two points about 2 cm apart by the thickened papillary muscles and tendons; centrally and laterally to these points the valve margins are free, though the two lateral commissures soon become adherent. The central portion remains open because of the stream of blood going through it. This suggestion was illustrated by specimens and lantern slides. Questions were asked about the appearance of the valve in mitral incompetence and the gradual development of rheumatic affection of the heart valves. Dr de Navasquez said that what Mr Brock had said agreed with what was seen at post mortem. Dr Campbell thanked Mr Brock for his classic contribution and said that the surgical exploration of

The Heart Club

the heart valves could now be added to the methods of investigating heart disease.

Dr de Navasquez said that there was much material for study in the routine biopsies of lung and auricular appendix which were taken at operation. The blocks had been saved and would be available for anyone interested in them.[*] The investigation might be tedious but would be rewarding. The diagnosis of pulmonary artery changes was very difficult because in a section it was not really possible to tell whether the artery seen was a pulmonary or a bronchial artery. It was pointed out that the lingula should contain a definite branch of the pulmonary artery which could be traced if the section was cut parallel to the cut surface of the lung.

Dr Graham showed a specimen of an A.V. fistula of the lung. Dr Starkey showed the specimen of a case which died suddenly after angiography. At post mortem it was thought that the catheter, through which the contrast medium was injected, must have been in the coronary sinus and not in the right ventricle. When compared with the angiocardiography picture it seemed likely that the catheter had in fact been in the right ventricular outflow tract at the time of injection, and that the radio-opaque material had burst through the myocardium and around the coronary sinus.

Specimens from Fish, and Gallagher were shown. The meeting closed at the late hour of 11.00 pm.

Feb 11th 1952
Maurice Campbell

---

* This invitation was taken up and several publications ensued. [73-75]

February 1952
At a meeting of the Peacock Club in the Wardens House on February 11th, 1952 there were present 11 members.

The date of the next meeting was fixed for March 17th, when acute rheumatic activity in adults will be discussed.

Dr Deuchar spoke on the cardiovascular pressures in congenital heart disease.[*] He first reviewed the catheterisation of congenital heart disease during the past year. He had found that if a catheter passed from the right ventricle to the aorta, pulmonary atresia was to be expected. Experience was enabling one to judge the site of the pulmonary stenosis, whether valvar or infundibular, to be judged more accurately at catheterisation.

The form of the arterial pressure pulse was described and the factors which influence its form considered. The resistance to the emptying of the ventricle was in part the arteriolar resistance and in part the elastic resistance of the arterial wall. Both these resistances can be calculated. It must be understood that the physical concept of elasticity differs from the popular one and may be defined by the formula K/V where K is an expression of the rigidity of the vessel wall and V is the volume of the arterial system. This formula indicates that a large arterial volume is associated with a low elasticity. The peripheral resistance of the systemic circulation is 7 times that of the pulmonary circulation but the elastic resistance of the vessels is only 2 ½ times that of the pulmonary vessels.

In primary pulmonary hypertension both peripheral and elastic resistance in the pulmonary circulation are increased and there is also a small increase in resistance in the systemic circulation. In Fallots Tetralogy there is an increase in the elastic resistance but the peripheral resistance of the systemic circulation is normal. In pulmonary stenosis the elastic resistance is low. In many cases the peripheral resistance of the pulmonary circulation is related to the clinical disability- presumably because of the organic changes in the lung vessels, though admittedly existing pathological methods cannot show these changes. Mr Brock here asked whether the speaker considered that

---

[*] This material was published by Dr Deuchar with Dr Zak and Dr Knebel in papers in Guys Hospital Reports and the *BHJ*.[76-78]

The Heart Club

the post stenotic pulmonary dilation was a primary condition or secondary to the stenosis. Had he considered that there might be constriction of the pulmonary vessels?

Dr Deuchar then showed the form of the ventricular pressure curve and considered the electrical analogy of the motive force and resistance in a number of conditions, especially in connection with the relation of resistance in the systemic circulation to that in the pulmonary circulation. He showed examples of right ventricular and pulmonary artery pressures taken at operation which were usually lower than those measured at catheterisation. After valvotomy in pulmonary stenosis a fall in right ventricular pressure occurs and a rise in pulmonary artery pressure. In Fallots Tetralogy the pressure pulse in the right ventricle and the infundibular chamber showing a step-like pulse of shorter duration than that in the right ventricle. The rise in pulmonary artery pressure after valvotomy in Fallots Tetralogy is often greater than in pulmonary stenosis. In one case the right to left ventricular shunt appeared to have been reversed by the operation.

Discussion on these points became general and the meeting continued until 23.05 hours.

March 17th 1952
Maurice Campbell

Tom Treasure

March 1952

A meeting of the Peacock Club was held on March 17th 1952, in the Wardens House. There were present 16 members. The date of the next meeting was undecided.

Dr Baker spoke of acute rheumatism* in patients with mitral stenosis. The success of valvotomy is likely to be affected by:

1. The condition of the valve.
2. The degree of myocardial involvement.
3. The presence of auricular fibrillation or cardiac failure.
4. The temperament of the patient.
5. Rheumatic activity.

Whether acute rheumatic activity is present is difficult to judge. If present it may be a serious hazard of both the immediate and the delayed post-operative period. Dr Baker then described the course of Brown and Garlick as an indication of the problem of acute rheumatic activity. The progress of Northey, Holdsworth, Nash, Hogarth and Gallagher, was described by Dr Venner, who emphasised the association of a pyrexial illness with progressive cardiac failure, and in one case there was joint involvement.

Dr Enticknap described the post mortem findings on Gallagher. In this and 40 other cases Aschoff nodes had not been found, but perhaps the left auricular appendix was not a hopeful place to find them. These findings did not correspond with those recently described in the *American Heart Journal*.

Mr Douglas asked about the possibility of treating these cases with A.C.T.H. and Cortisone. The danger of sodium retention was put forward against it.

Dr Bywaters said all his post mortem studies on acute rheumatic fever in children had shown Aschoff nodes in the heart, but the left auricular appendix had not been examined. He understood by rheumatic activity joint pains and tachycardia. The E.S.R. was raised and the Westergren was a better method than the Wintrobe. Serum fibrinogen studies might help.

---

* See acute rheumatism in the Glossary and also rheumatic fever.
  Dr Enticknap published this work in the *BHJ*.[73]

The Heart Club

Dr Starkey said that at the Bellevue Hospital the opinion was held that an Aschoff node did not denote activity.

The meeting closed at 11.08 hours.

October 27th 1952 Maurice Campbell

Tom Treasure

BRITISH MEDICAL JOURNAL

LONDON SATURDAY MAY 17 1952

VALVOTOMY FOR MITRAL STENOSIS

A FURTHER REPORT, ON 100 CASES

BY

CHARLES BAKER, M.D., F.R.C.P.   R. C. BROCK, M.S., F.R.C.S., F.A.C.S.(Hon.)

MAURICE CAMPBELL, D.M., F.R.C.P.

AND

PAUL WOOD, M.D., F.R.C.P.

(From Guy's Hospital, the Brompton Hospital, and the Institute of Cardiology)

Our interest in valvotomy for mitral stenosis extends back over several years, although it was not until September, 1948, that our first patient was operated on. In June, 1950, we were able to report our experiences in nine patients, seven with successful operations (Baker, Brock, and Campbell, 1950). We are now able to report the immediate results on 100 patients treated by operation, with a more detailed analysis and follow-up of the first 50, the last of whom was operated upon in May, 1951, so that all have been followed for six months, the majority for more than a year, and some for two to three years. Apart from two patients at the Johns Hopkins Hospital, Baltimore, the operations were done at either Guy's Hospital or the Brompton Hospital, and all by one surgeon. For the purpose of analysis and follow-up the two Baltimore cases have been omitted from the first 50.

In previous papers we have followed common usage in writing of pulmonary or mitral " valvulotomy," but it is a valve and not a valvule that is divided, and we think the term " valvotomy " is more correct, even though it is still a hybrid formation. The operation really does more than splitting the commissures, for if the valve cusps are reasonably supple the operation may enable them to close better and more normally, but we have thought it better to reserve the term " valvoplasty " for more elaborate operations that may be possible in the future.

Present Position of Mitral Valvotomy

Our earlier paper contained a fairly full presentation of the problem of mitral valvotomy up to that time, and there is no need for repetition here. The great improvement observed in seven of the nine patients enabled us to say with some confidence that the operative relief of mitral stenosis was a practical procedure with a reasonably low mortality, and that it could justifiably be recommended in suitable cases and would probably have a wider application. Our subsequent experience reported here with 100 cases and with 32 good or excellent results in the follow-up of the first 50, as well as the experience of several other clinics, amply confirms these views.

The relatively low mortality of the operation deserves immediate emphasis. Thus of our first 20 patients, 7 died ; only one more patient died in the next 30, making 8 deaths in the first 50 cases, and only 5 more in the next 50, making 13 deaths in the first 100 cases. Even severely ill patients with advanced mitral stenosis will stand cardiotomy well, *provided the mechanical obstruction within the heart is relieved by the operation.*

As soon as our first report appeared the great need for operative relief of mitral stenosis was borne vividly upon us by the large number of patients presenting themselves for consideration, the requests coming from cardiologists, from general practitioners, and from the patients themselves. A future that previously seemed bleak for many patients, generally under 40 and often under 30 years of age, has been completely changed. It is only in dealing with a large number of these patients that one realizes the true extent of the tragedies that mitral stenosis can produce.

Successful surgical treatment of mitral stenosis has disclosed a problem of great extent. Congenital heart lesions, for instance, constitute only 2% of all cases of heart disease, and it is fair to say that their operative relief is best undertaken in a few special centres. By contrast, rheumatism causes 25% of cases of heart disease in hospital (Wood, 1950), and in half of them mitral stenosis is the predominant lesion. It is not possible for all the patients for whom operation is required to be dealt with in a few special centres. Mitral valvotomy is now a standard procedure that should be practised in all thoracic surgical clinics in large centres.

Although a new field of surgery has been opened up, the problem is even larger than the purely surgical conception. In some respects it is comparable with that of pulmonary tuberculosis, in which surgery has come to play a large and increasing part, but is still only one factor in the general management. Many patients with mitral stenosis, as many with pulmonary tuberculosis, will never need operation, but must have medical treatment. Close co-operation between surgeon and physician is essential, and when operation is needed the selection of the best time for surgery comes from

4767

The publication of the first 100 mitral valvotomy operations in the British Medical Journal.[118]

The Heart Club

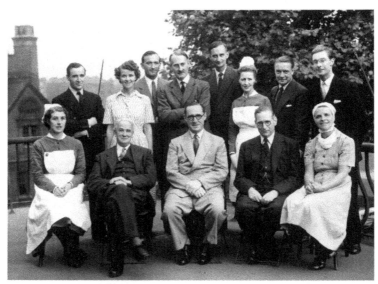

Dr Campbell, Mr Brock and Dr Rink are central, flanked by two theatre nurses. Behind are Peter Fleming, Chris Jones (Brocks secretary), Ben Milstein, Charles Baker, an unnamed doctor and nurse, Eddie Holling and Ian Hill. The photograph was taken to celebrate the 100th Brock procedure and the operating room scene is below. Brock and Dr Rink are recognizable despite their masks and the nurses seem to be the two in the group photograph taken on the roof. Pictures provided by Alison Hill and the Gordon Museum.

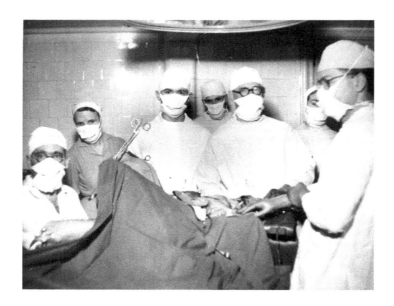

October 1952

There was a meeting of the Peacock Club in the Staff Common Room at 8.15 pm on October 27th 1952. Seven members were present.

Dr Deuchar showed pathological specimens of congenital heart disease.

Mr Brunnen then described experiences with experimental aortic grafting.* Clearly in the case of the aorta venous grafts are not a practical proposition and grafts of synthetic materials are liable to rupture. Aortic homografts were introduced in 1948.

Such grafts are difficult to obtain. They should be obtained from young people within 6 to 10 hours of death, but to do this at present introduces legal difficulties; the coroner must be acquiescent. For such purposes sterile equipment must be kept always ready. The bank can seldom keep a large stock of grafts on hand.

Various methods of keeping grafts are available. The favoured method is to freeze the vessels rapidly at -20°C and then to store at 0 to 4°C in a balanced electrolyte solution.

Tissue drying at low temperature is under trial.

It is important, however, to solve the problem of how to sterilize grafts which could not be taken under conditions of optimum sterility. Electron beam sterilization at low temperature appears to sterilise without tissue damage. Formalin 4% as a sterilizing agent appears of use.

After transplantation host tissues grow into the graft. A new intima is fairly quickly deposited but elastic media is more slowly changed (About 3 years).

In animal experiments at Guys 8 dogs were grafted with grafts aseptically obtained, frozen in CO snow and kept in deep freeze. Six were sacrificed and excellent results found in 4, good in 2.

---

* Mr Brunnen published this work in Guys Hospital Reports.[79]
See homograft in the Glossary.

The Heart Club

Seven dogs had grafts which had been obtained without sterile precautions and subsequently irradiated by cathode ray at -20°C. (To prevent tissue destruction it seems important to give the dose rate as quickly as possible, 1 10^{-6} sec. possibly.

Of these 7 cases, 4 (dose 75 sec.), thrombosed and ruptured, 3 (dose 15 secs.) thrombosed, 1 had a good result.

Of 3 cases treated with formalin 4%, 1 thrombosed and 2 had good results, but formalin treated material is technically difficult to use. Of 3 cases treated with formalin 48 hours and then frozen, 1 thrombosed, 1 had an excellent result and in one the result is still not known. One graft 10 months old kept in balanced salt solution was friable and partial thrombosis took place.

Specimens of grafts were shown.

The date of the next meeting was provisionally decided as November 25th, the subject for discussion to be Pulmonary Changes in Mitral Stenosis to be opened by Dr Baker and Dr Enticknap.

November 25th 1952
Maurice Campbell

November 1952

A meeting of the Peacock Club was held in Dr Bakers house at 8.15 pm. on Tuesday, November 25th 1952. There were 14 members present and by invitation Dr R. Gorlin of Boston.

The date of the next meeting was fixed for January 13th, 1953, the subject to be Congenital Heart Disease, and the opening speaker, Dr Campbell.

Dr Enticknap described the changes in the lingula biopsies taken from cases of mitral stenosis.* Gross obliteration of the main vessel might occur and organic thrombi were found in one-sixth of the vessels. Obliterative endarteritis was, however, rare. Perivenous fibrosis was sometimes seen but the importance of it was not known. Occasionally fibrinoid lesions were seen in the media which were similar to those lesions described in malignant systemic hypertension, but since they did not occur in cases with the highest pulmonary artery pressure it seemed unlikely that they were due to hypertension. The hyaline changes of systemic hypertension were not seen.

More than one-third of the cases showed hypertrophy of the pulmonary arterioles; this is measured in terms of the ratio of thickness of the wall to that of the lumen; a ratio of 2 to 1 indicates hypertrophy. Hypertrophy of the pulmonary arterioles was found to be related to the mean pulmonary artery pressure.

The distribution of haemosiderosis in the lungs of mitral stenosis was then shown in whole lung sections. This occurred in the upper parts of the lobes, and the lingula appeared to be free. The lingula did, however, show haemosiderosis on section. In sections haemosiderin was found to be accumulated in phagocytes within the lumen of the alveoli.

Dr Baker then showed X-Rays of patients with mitral stenosis and haemosiderosis. He had classed the degree of haemosiderosis into 4 grades though he stressed that this grading was very subjective. Of 33 cases 6 showed Grade 3 mottling of the lungs, 7 Grade 2, and 8 showed no mottling. The x-ray appearances differ from those of pulmonary congestion because the shadows are hard and the appearance is mottled. Marked haemosiderosis

---

* Dr Enticknap published this work in the *Journal of Clinical Pathology*.[74]

The Heart Club

may be seen though there is no history of haemoptyses, and the pulmonary artery pressure is not unduly elevated.

The degree of haemosiderosis seen on x-ray and that seen in sections only slightly correspond. In any case it seems that the combination of x-rays and catheter show all that a biopsy could.

Mr Milstein pointed out the possible dangers of doing a lung biopsy, for cases having had a biopsy had higher and longer post operative pyrexia, required more pleural aspiration and showed a shadow in the region of the biopsy.

Mr Brock pointed out the selective incidence of the segments affected by haemosiderosis and suggested that this might be due to haemorrhage from bronchi; but if it is due to haemorrhage, why no haemoptysis? Mr Brain thought it unlikely that the force of gravity could account for the distribution. Dr Hills spoke on the technical aspects of x-raying and interpreting haemosiderosis. Dr Gorlin reported that Dr Suzman found haemosiderosis and vascular congestion hard to distinguish. He remarked that changes in histological section did not correlate with physiological findings but did with x-ray.

Mr Ian Hill thought the techniques of biopsy was improving and wondered if the linear pattern seen more clearly in mitrals was due to lymphatics.

The meeting closed at 10.30 p.m.

R.C. Brock
13.1.53

Tom Treasure

January 1953

At a meeting of the Peacock Club on January 13th, 1953 there were present 13 members. The date of the next meeting was fixed as Tuesday, February 17th, when pathological specimens are to be shown. Mr Milstein accepted the duty of Secretary during Dr Hollings absence abroad.

Dr Campbell then spoke on the natural history of congenital heart disease. More than 1,000 cases had been observed, of which 60% were cyanosed and 40% acyanosed. The natural incidence of cyanotic heart disease was probably higher.

There were 5 roughly equal groups of acyanotic cases, P.D.A., V.S.D., A.S.D., P.V.S., and classed together Aortic Stenosis and Coarctation.* Of the cyanotic group two-thirds were Fallots Tetralogy, rather less than 10% were cases of pulmonary atresia of which one half had a continuous murmur and a good prognosis, and one half no murmur and a poorer prognosis.

Fewer cases with transposition were seen than if this series had included children under 5. Whereas this malformation carries a poor prognosis, that associated (perhaps unjustly) with Eisenmengers name has a good prognosis. No coarctation over 40 was seen, nor were older patients with P.D.A. seen. In post mortem experience cerebral abscess was frequent as a cause of death, bacterial endocarditis rare. Seven of the eight cases of atrial septal defect who died were beyond middle age. No P.D.As or Coarctations were seen at post mortem; possibly they die younger. The mortality among the cases of P.V.S. appeared to be high.

The figures showed how much more killing cyanotic heart disease was than acyanotic. The prognosis of tricuspid atresia appeared to be greatly improved by operation. Congenital aortic stenosis may be difficult to diagnose and is often associated with no limitation of activity.

Mr Brain asked about the differential diagnosis of truncus and pulmonary atresia and whether patients with cyanotic heart disease were fertile.

---

* See coarctation in the Glossary.

THE INCIDENCE OF CONGENITAL HEART DISEASE

	M/F
Acyanotic Heart Disease	
Coarctation	3/2
Aortic stenosis	3/1
P.D.A.	2/3
A.S.D.	Equal.
V.S.D.	"
P.V.S.	"
A.S.D. (over 25)	5/1
Cyanotic Heart Disease	
Fallot's Tetralogy }	3/2
Transposition }	
Eisenmenger	2/1

MORTALITY OF ANNUAL & MORTALITY OF CASES

A.S.D.	1%	(raised to 15% if infants & older patients; 3 over 60 are included.
P.D.A.	2%	(5% with other systemic pulmonary fistula)
P.V.S.	3%	
Cyanotic		
Pulmonary atresia	40	
T. atresia }	30	
Transposition of vessels }		
P.V.S. with P.T.O. (cyanotic)	20	
Fallot's Tetralogy	10	

Table 1 for the January 1953 meeting.

Tom Treasure

CLASSIFICATION OF 460 CASES OF
ACYANOTIC CONGENITAL HEART DISEASE

			Percentage
Aortic stenosis	32		7
Coarctation of aorta	52	84	11.5
V.V.S. (including 2 with infundibular stenosis and 5 with left to right shunts as well).		74	16.5
P.D.A. (including 7 with other aortico-pulmonary communications and 1 with P.D.A. on right).		104	22
A.S.D. (including 1 with V.V.S. and 5 with anomalous pulmonary veins draining into R. atrium)		81	18
V.S.D. (including 2 with P.V.S. and 1 with a right sided aortic arch).		99	21
Unclassified (including 5 with dextrocardia).		18	4
		460	100%

CLASSIFICATION OF 670 CASES OF
CYANOTIC CONGENITAL HEART DISEASE

			Percentage
Fallot's tetralogy (including 4 with a single ventricle		385	57
Pulmonary atresia - Fallot + atresia	32		
with continuous murmur	27	59	9
Transposition		56	8
P.V.S. with R.S.D		42	6
Eisenmenger's complex		42	6
Tricuspid atresia		31	5
Dextrocardia and laevocardia		31	5
Unclassified (including 5 with Ebstein's disease).		24	4
		670	100

Feb 1st 1953   Maurice Campbell

Table 2 for the January 1953 meeting.

The Heart Club

Dr Deuchar pointed out that increased pulmonary blood flow as in A.S.D. may be associated with poor oxygenation in alveoli.

Mr Brock stressed the danger of cerebral abscess in Fallots Tetralogy and said he did not like to operate on cases over 20, but had to do so if they had low infundibular stenosis. He thought that the figures from Bristol were unreliable. P.D.A. may not have a continuous murmur and is often misdiagnosed.

Feb 17th 1953
Maurice Campbell

February 1953

A meeting of the Peacock Club was held on 17th February 1953 in the Gordon Museum. 17 members were present and, by invitation, Dr Ian McMillan of St Thomass Hospital.

The date of the next meeting was fixed as Tuesday 24th March, when Dr Hills would show some unusual angiocardiograms and open a discussion on their interpretation.

Dr McMillan showed some films of movements of normal and pathological heart valves.* In an advanced case of rheumatic aortic stenosis, he pointed out that the peripheral third of the commissure was heavily calcified and not amenable to splitting. He then showed the movements of the aortic valve in the case of Denny (aortic stenosis) after valvotomy. There was some discussion about the size of the orifice and the direction of the split.

Dr McMillan then showed films of the mitral valve. The first was of a normal valve. The aortic cusp could be seen to be responsible for most of the movement. He then showed the valve in a case of tight mitral stenosis before and after valvotomy. At first the movement of the cusps is slight and the chordae move more than the cusps themselves, but after valvotomy the movement of the aortic cusp is much increased.

There were a number of questions on the technique of preparation of the specimens and cinematography.

Dr Campbell said that he thought that many more of the cases of aortic stenosis then it was usually believed were of congenital origin. He thought that both Denny and Littler were examples of congenital aortic stenosis and that many of the calcified atherosclerotic valves were congenital.

Dr Deuchar then showed a series of pathological specimens as follows:

Denny and Littler – Aortic stenosis: Death following valvotomy.

---

* This was further work in progress published in 1955.[80]

The Heart Club

Phoebe Thomas – Mitral stenosis and tricuspid stenosis: Acute pulmonary oedema after catheterisation.

Dr Enticknap showed sections of the lungs from this case:

Veronica Bell – Subacute bacterial endocarditis due to Ps. Pyocyanea following mitral valvotomy. It was observed that the main vegetation was at the site of incision in the medical commissure.

Basil Rochford – Pulmonary valvular stenosis with an A.S.D. and a low V.S.D. and abnormal muscle bundles in the right ventricular outflow tract. This patient died following upper right lobectomy for an aspergillus abscess.

Rose Rockett – Fallots Tetralogy treated by infundibular resection and valvotomy. Aneurysm of the right ventricle at the site of the cardiotomy compressing the pulmonary artery. Valvotomy had divided one cusp and perforated another.

Pearl Thorpe – Fallots Tetralogy treated by Blalock operation.* Sudden death from acute pulmonary oedema, in spite of perfect result at two-year follow up.

Joan Price – Fallots Tetralogy treated by infundibular resection. Death from ascending myelitis 9 months after operation. The infundibular stenosis was seen to have been completely relieved.

Two cases of truncus arteriosus. In one of these the pulmonary arteries arose from a single trunk leaving the aorta. In the other case two separate pulmonary arteries arose from the aorta.

Mr Hill showed the following cases:

Eustace- Mitral valvotomy. Death from pyopneumothorax 6 weeks after operation.

---

* See Blalock operation in the Glossary.

Tom Treasure

A case of Fallots Tetralogy treated by Blalock operation in which death had occurred after 3 hours. Both valvular and infundibular stenosis were present.

Dr Enticknap showed sections of the heart and lungs from some of these cases.

The meeting closed at 10.45 pm.

March 24th 1953
Maurice Campbell

The Heart Club

March 1953

A meeting of the Peacock Club was held on Tuesday 24th March, in the Gordon Museum. 8 members were present.

Dr Hills showed series of angiocardiograms from the following cases:

1. Frost: Clinically this appeared to be a case of Fallots Tetralogy. The left ventricular preponderance was thought to be due to the position of the heart. At operation by Mr Holmes Sellors, two superior venae cavae were found. The right one was said to enter the right atrium and the left one the left atrium. The left superior vena cava was ligated and a Blalock operation performed. Subsequently the child died.

    Post mortem diagnosis: There was practically a single atrium with a single A.V. valve and a single ventricle. The left superior vena cava was closely applied to the pulmonary veins. The angiocardiogram did not show the presence of the single atrium or ventricle. It did, however, indicate the presence of an infundibular chamber.

2. Diana Bevan: The angiocardiogram showed a double superior vena cava, the left one apparently entering the coronary sinus. There was gross over-riding of the aorta. The pulmonary arteries were well filled at 2 seconds. This patient had a continuous murmur and the question arose as to whether the pulmonary arteries were filling from a patent ductus or a patent pulmonary trunk. Dr Campbell said that clinically the diagnosis was pulmonary atresia with a ductus.

    Mr Hill said that a main pulmonary artery was present and that there would have been better filling in the 1½ seconds film if a ductus had been present.

    Dr Deuchar suggested that there might be a bronchial artery joining the pulmonary artery.

    Dr Hills pointed out that the diodone had just entered the abdominal aorta at the same time as filling of the main pulmonary arteries commenced. This suggested a patent ductus.

3. Diana Pearce: The angiocardiograms showed a right superior vena cava and a left superior vena cava entering the coronary sinus. There was a right sided over-riding aorta but this did not fill as well as the pulmonary artery. Both trunks filled from the right ventricle. A round shadow could be seen around the pulmonary artery.

Tom Treasure

Mr Hill suggested that this was a ductus which was closed at its aortic end as he had seen a similar case.

Dr Hills thought that it was the main pulmonary artery projecting upwards above its branches.

Dr Campbell was observing this child and said that he would recommend operation if there were no improvement.

4. Pether: The clinical condition suggested Fallots Tetralogy but there was left ventricular preponderance. The angiocardiogram appeared to indicate transposition of the great vessels with pulmonary stenosis.

   Dr Deuchar suggested that it was a case of tricuspid atresia with transposition and pulmonary stenosis. The aortic arch curved to the right but descended on the left and there was some discussion as to whether this should be called a left or right arch.

5. Mather: In this case the stomach was on the right and the liver more on the right than the left.

   Both Dr Campbell and Mr Hill pointed out that as there was a diminished pulmonary blood flow and an early right-to-left shunt, this patient was at any rate suitable for treatment by anastomosis.

   Mr Hill thought that a large atrial septal defect might be present.

6. Angel: This case had been diagnosed as Fallots Tetralogy. It was clear that pulmonary valvular stenosis was present but the right ventricle was very small.

   Dr Campbell thought that it was too small for a case of Fallots Tetralogy. It was remarked that the left atrium appeared to fill in the ½ second film and in fact the operative diagnosis was pulmonary valvular stenosis with atrial septal defect.

7. Pike: This was a case of transposition of the great vessels with pulmonary stenosis, proved at operation. There was a good result following a Blalock operation.

8. Huson: The angiocardiogram showed pulmonary atresia with an enormous right bronchial artery. There were no pulmonary arteries.

   Dr Deuchar suggested that a bronchial artery fills from the descending aorta. There was also an abdominal aortic branch to the left lung.

9. Dant: The segment below the left subclavian artery was seen to be short and another vessel arose immediately proximal to the left subclavian.

   Mr Hill thought that the picture did not suggest that the conditions

The Heart Club

were unfavourable for operative treatment. He suggested that the proximal vessel was part of a double left subclavian artery.

10. Waugh: This was a case of Fallots Tetralogy. There was some discussion as to whether the stenosis was valvular or high infundibular. Mr Hill thought that it was double.

11. Richards: From the angiocardiographic point of view, this appeared to be a case of transposition of the great vessels and atrial septal defect, who subsequently became cyanosed. A shadow on the plain film in the left upper chest did not fill with diodone and the angiocardiogram gave no help in eliciting it.

    Dr Campbell suggested that this was the picture of pulmonary veins draining into a left superior vena cava.

12. Collins: This was a case of isolated dextrocardia with pleonaemic lungs. Catheterisation showed a shunt into a right atrium. The angiocardiograms suggested pulmonary veins draining into the right atrium. The aorta descended on the right and there were large pulmonary arteries. The great vessels appeared to arise from the right ventricle.

    Dr Campbell pointed out that our diagnosis skill in interpreting angiocardiograms had not increased much on account of the very difficult cases which were now being presented for diagnostic.

The meeting closed at 10.30 pm. November 19th 1953 Maurice Campbell*

---

* The minutes signed a couple of weeks after the next meeting.

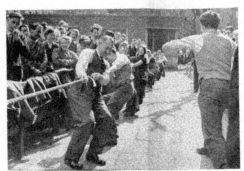

Dr. Baker leads Dr. Boland's Firm.

Mr. Doherty, in his capacity as Superintendent and Umpire, then presented Dr. Baker, as leader of the winning side, with the cup amid scenes of considerable enthusiasm. So ended a pleasant afternoon and the revival of yet another old Guy's custom.

D.B.L.   C.B.

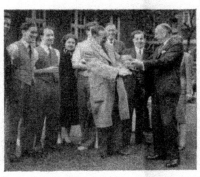

The Superintendent congratulates Dr. Boland on retaining the Davies-Colley Cup.

TEAMS :

Dr. Boland's Firm :
Dr. C. G. Baker, Dr. K. MacLean, Dr. D. Deuchar, Dr. P. Dunbar, Mr. C. Bishop, Miss G. H. Cann, Mr. A. E. Kenmuir-Evans, Mr. D. B. Longmore, Mr. E. Moran, Miss J. Platnaur, Mr. M. D. Vickers and Mr. K. Wilderspin.

Sir John Conybeare's Firm :—
Mr. K. Lee, Mr. J. Greeves, Mr. I. Macdougall, Mr. D. Miller, Miss D. Collins, Mr. Y. Nalletamby, Mr. A. Aistrop, Miss May Jaques, Mr. H. Carling, Mr. I. Reid, Dr. B. Tudgay, Dr. J. Smith, Dr. K. Gray and Dr. T. Finnegan.

Interviewed after the contest, a member of Dr. Boland's firm commented as follows : " I couldn't have pulled much longer "— his face tightened, " Oh my hamstrings ! " This is regarded as substantial evidence of the quality of the tractive effort expended by Sir John's narrowly defeated team.

(Photographs by kind permission of Fox Photos Ltd.)

Tug of War from Guys Hospital Gazette May 1953. Charles Baker captained the winning team for Dr Bolands firm which included Dennis Deuchar and a medical student Jane Platnaur. She was later Brocks resident 1955/6 and married Walter Somerville. She can be seen in both photographs. See Biographical Notes for further information.

The Heart Club

November 1953
A meeting of the Club took place at 8.15 pm in the Gordon Museum and the Wardens House on November 3rd.

There were present 12 members and Dr Kittle of Kansas. Pathological specimens were shown. One of Mr Hill was an M.S. 6/12 after valvotomy. The date of the next meeting was fixed for Tues Dec 8th when Mr Ross will speak on Hypothermia.

Dr Holling spoke on his visit to USA.

In Philadelphia he worked with Dr Starr on the Ballistocardiograph.*

It was an inferior way of measuring cardiac output and is now regarded as a measurement of cardiac force. 4,000 are in use in the USA, it is useful for the management of coronary disease. He also worked with Lysle Peterson on measurement of acceleration of blood along the aorta using a dye injection technique and a cuvette. With Dr Hugh Montgomery he measured the oxygen tension of muscle with a platinum electrode.

He spoke of Sawyer and Pates work on the injury current in arterial grafts and its effects on thrombosis. This work suggests that it would be better to use dead than living grafts. If the graft is insulated with mineral oil there is less thrombosis.

At the meeting of vascular surgeons in the New York in May, the wrapping of arterial grafts had been discussed. At the M.G.H. Boston arteriograms were frequently employed and the saphenous vein grafted into the femoral artery. In discussion the danger of arterial thrombosis with diodine was mentioned, Dr Campbell mentioned the danger of angina in relieving claudication.

In upper limb sympathectomy a ganglionectomy is now done, but the reason why lower limb sympathectomy is so much more satisfactory than upper limb is not understood.

---

* See ballistocardiography in the Glossary.
  See sympathectomy and ganglionectomy.

Tom Treasure

Cardiac Output
Cournands insistence on the importance of the steady state. Fick Principle*

Mr Hill and Dr Campbells opinion was that great accuracy was not required for clinical purposes.

The dye injection method is largely used and can be quickly done but determinations cannot be repeated otherwise patient is dyed blue. Blue is also difficult to see against cyanotic blood.

Alternative method is to use radioactive indicator in blood, something which sticks in blood stream is desirable.

The dye method is also used for detection of shunts in congenital heart disease.

Harkens method of dealing with mitral incompetence by means of a plastic prosthesis was discussed. The surgeon is enthusiastic the physicians less so. In Sept 24 cases had been operated on with 7 deaths, 11 survived 2 years 5 greatly improved.

Hufnagel (Washington D.C.) has been putting a plastic non return valve in the aorta for aortic incompetence. 1 death in last 10 cases. Do well but Dr Baker remarks that these cases do well until failure.

Potts (Chicago) favoured shunt operation for pulmonary stenosis because mortality lower (in his hands).

Crafoord questioned whether Eisenmenger might develop.

Dr Campbell saw only one patient had increased pressure, this is important not pressure. Mr Hill had had one case at Barts pulmonary plethora.

---

* See Fick principle in the Glossary.
  See dye in the Glossary.
  St Bartholomews Hospital.

The Heart Club

Dr Holling said there was great interest in the comparison between direct and indirect operations on Fallots Tetralogy.

The meeting closed at 11.05 pm.

December 8th 1953
Maurice Campbell

Tom Treasure

December 1953

A meeting of the Peacock Club was held at 8.00 pm on December 8th 1953, in the Pathology Department. 21 members were present.

The next meeting was arranged for Tuesday, February 2nd, 1954, the subject to be decided.

Mr Ross demonstrated apparatus in the Animal Operating Room and then spoke on his experiences with experimental hypothermia* in dogs. The object of hypothermia is to provide opportunity for cardiac operations without the complications of an artificial lung. Cooling may be from the surface or internally by including a cooling device in the circulation.

Morphine, grains 1/6th and Atropine grains 1/100th are given followed by pentothal and perhaps ether and oxygen. Neither quinidine nor procaine is required. Blood from the femoral artery is passed into the femoral vein through 9 feet of Portex tubing immersed in cold brine. The system contains 50 ml. blood. In about an hour the body temperature falls to 25°C. Below this temperature cardiac abnormalities are frequent. At this temperature the pulse is about 60/min., the blood pressure 80 mm Hg and respiration may or may not continue. Rewarming is better done by moderate external warmth but may be done by using the cooling coil as a warming coil.

The circulation can be stopped for 5 to 7 minutes and for longer if the coronaries are perfused by blood injected into the aorta. When superior and inferior venae cavae are clamped the right atrium collapses and may prolapse into the ventricle and the ventricular rhythm is disturbed. The mortality of such operations is about 30%.

Physiological investigations show that the clotting time is prolonged but returns to normal when the blood is warmed. The blood pressure falls and the formation of urine also.

Oxygen consumption falls with the temperature.

---

* See hypothermia in the Glossary.
This work was published in Guys Hospital Reports and in *The Lancet*.[81-83]
Pentothal is an anaesthetic agent.

The E.C.G. shows widened and notched QRS and the T is inverted. There is haemoconcentration. Blood potassium is lowered and the pH falls to 6.9 but may be put back to normal by hyperventilating.

It is still not clear whether surface or blood stream cooling is better. Below 27°C no anaesthesia is required. The cardiac irregularities are increased by cyclopropane* but this is probably due to increased CO. Some workers produce ventricular fibrillation purposely to reduce the oxygen requirements of the heart.

Dr Campbell thanked Mr Ross for his able presentation.

Dr Jouvenelle [sic] (Paris) said that experiments showed that renal function as shown by diodrast clearance or bromosulphothalein excretion falls with the fall of temperature. Barbiturates may be dangerous in hypothermia and become fixed in the brain for he found that one dog was showing the effects of barbiturate poisoning for 7 days. He favoured rapid rewarming.

He pressed the need for basic research to find out, for example, how hibernating animals differed from normal animals. He also pointed out how measurements of blood electrolytes did not tell what was happening in the cells; making the simile that we found what was happening in the streets but did not know what was occurring in the houses.

The cardiac muscle is effective in removing oxygen from the blood stream and does not suffer in fibrillation. Fibrillation may prevent air embolism.

Mr Brock pointed out that the human heart seemed to withstand fibrillation better than the dog heart.

Dr Hutton said that under operative conditions it was difficult to hyperventilate the patient so that there was a real chance of the acid base balance being upset.

---

* See cyclopropane in the Glossary.
 Believed to be André Juvenelle who was working on hypothermia in Paris.[84]

Tom Treasure

Dr Baker asked whether the practice of cooling psychiatric patients had produced any information of value. Dr Jouvenelle [sic] spoke of patients being at 24 to 27°c for days. They were semiconscious.

In conclusion Mr Ross again spoke of the danger of rapid rewarming.

The meeting closed at 10.35 p.m.

Feb 9th 1954
Maurice Campbell

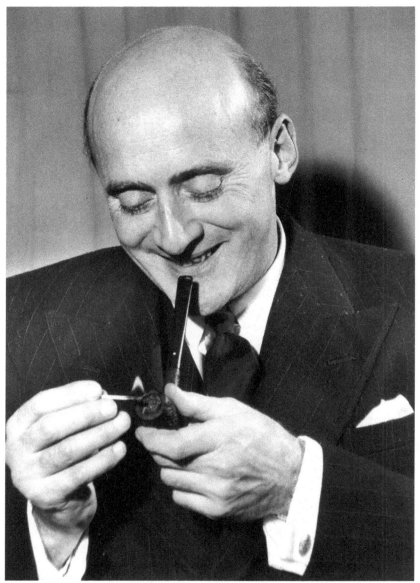

Mike Hutton (1916–1980) was a regular anaesthetist for cardiothoracic surgery and spoke at the meetings in December 1953 and February 1954.

Tom Treasure

February 1954

A meeting of the Peacock Club was held in the staff Common Room on February 9th, 1954. There were present 21 members.

The next meeting was arranged for Tuesday, March 9th, the speakers to be Dr Venner and Dr Shepherd [sic].* The subject to be decided.

Mr Milstein spoke on Ventricular Fibrillation. He sketched in a historical background to his talk showing that from the early days of chloroform anaesthesia ventricular fibrillation had been recognised. It must now be expected as an incident which may arise at any time during operations on the myocardium. Our methods of dealing with it are continuously improving. This is shown by the finding that of 11 cases of ventricular fibrillation which occurred at Guys between 1947 and 1952 only 1 recovered, whereas of the 10 cases occurring in 1953, 5 recovered. Ventricular fibrillation had also occurred during cardiac catheterisation, though not at this hospital. In the literature, which seldom included fatal cases, 8 cases had recovered after cardiac massage, 5 after electric defibrillation aided by procaine.

The recognition of ventricular fibrillation may be by electrocardiogram, or when the pericardium is open, by seeing the fibrillation. S-T depression and bundle branch block in the electrocardiogram may be forerunners of fibrillation. Precipitating factors are myocardial anoxia, carbon dioxide retention, and marked changes in pH. These conditions may suddenly arise when the outflow tract of the heart is obstructed. Whether cyclopropane or intravenous drugs predispose is uncertain. Hearts which are hypertrophied appear to be more irritable and therefore liable to fibrillate, and are more difficult to treat.

---

* Known to be Roy Jesse Shephard. He published numerous papers related to his work at Guys.[85-97] In an email to me in January 2017 he wrote Yes, I am the guilty party, although as so often around the world my name was listed as Shepherd rather than Shephard. It is an uncommon variant of a common name. That having been verified, subsequent uses of Shepherd have therefore been changed to Shephard.

Milstein published on ventricular fibrillation in cardiac surgery in Guys Hospital Reports.[98]

The Heart Club

Adrenaline may predispose to fibrillation which used in the absence of asystole. Diodone may result in conditions which favour the fibrillation. Coronary disease and coronary air embolism favour development of the condition.

Treatment is by cardiac massage and adequate pulmonary ventilation. Pulmonary ventilation does not invariably require intubation for a face mask may suffice. When cardiac massage is attempted an anterior thoracotomy should be done for transdiaphragmatic massage is less effective than direct massage.

Both hands should be used, for a large heart may be difficult to compress. A pause between squeezes should be allowed for cardiac filling. Too firm massage is likely to damage the myocardium. Procaine is the most effective of available drugs though when it fails electrical defibrillation has been known to succeed.*

Adrenaline is employed and also calcium chloride.

In electrical defibrillation the entire myocardium is put into the refractory phase in the hope that normal rhythm may then re-establish itself. Well padded electrodes are required to obviate danger of electrical burns.

Dr Campbell thanked Dr Milstein.

Mr Brock spoke of the alteration of attitude to this condition with the recognition that active measures can overcome it. Electrical defibrillation is not necessary but attention to maintenance of myocardial tone and coronary flow are. Only recently have patients with myocardial disease recovered once they have fibrillated.

Dr Rink was of the opinion that the main predisposing cause of ventricular fibrillation was a clinically serious cardiac condition. It was unlikely that

---

* See John Hunts personal account in this book. He is one of the three blue babies who tells his story in the next chapter. He was probably the first patient to have external defibrillation, administered by Donald Ross. [99]

the anaesthetist interrupted insufflations on any occasion for more than 30 seconds. Cyclopropane did not cause fibrillation if properly used.

Dr Hutton thought that cyclopropane did predispose the heart to fibrillation. When the condition was developed all measures to aid the circulation, including tilting the table should be used. Massage of the heart was better than electrical defibrillation.

Mr Hill thought it difficult to recognise ventricular fibrillation with certainty. Local damage to the heart is undoubtedly a factor in its causation. He was not certain that adrenaline was curative but it was often the drug given last before fibrillation was cured.

Dr Shephard questioned the statement that the carbon dioxide content could double during a period of an anaesthetists inattention to insufflation; this implied a carbon dioxide production of more than 10 times the normal.

Though Dr Venner did not consider it of practical importance to distinguish between fibrillation and tachycardia he doubted our capacity to do so.

Mr Milstein thought it unlikely that local trauma would give rise to fibrillation. Procaine seemed an effective curative drug. Cyclopropane should be used with caution because changes may progress though administration had been stopped. He thought that the most serious phase was when the myocardium was involved in fine movements, coarser movements were a stage of less serious import.

The meeting closed at 10.40 p.m.

R.C. Brock
March 16th 1954

The Heart Club

March 1954

A meeting of the Peacock Club took place on March 16th, 1954 in Dr Bakers House. There were present 11 members.

Tuesday, May 4th was suggested as the date of the next meeting when pathological specimens would be shown and Mr Brock would speak on the surgery of Aortic Stenosis.

Dr Shephard then spoke on the pulmonary blood flow and pressures in cases with a left to right shunt. His remarks were based on the findings in 24 cases of P.D.A., 17 of A.S.D. and 14 of V.S.D.[*] In some of these patients it was admittedly difficult to get satisfactory figures for the pulmonary blood flow. The criteria of diagnosis in the different cases was discussed and the terms used explained.

In 10 cases of P.D.A. the pulmonary systolic pressure was normal; in the others but slightly increased; the diastolic was usually raised. There was a typical pulse tracing in the ductus itself. In the cases of A.S.D. the systolic pressure was higher though the diastolic might be less than in P.D.A. In V.S.D. the pressure is influenced by the left ventricular pressure and the pulmonary pulse pressure tends to be wide.

In all three conditions a pressure gradient at the pulmonary valve may occur. This was sometimes called a relative stenosis but its true nature was not known.

The mean flow in all three groups of cases was similar, i.e. 2.4 to 2.8 times the normal flow, and tended to be less when the pressure was above 100 mm Hg.

Pulmonary pressures seemed to be higher in the older patients especially those with A.S.D. Increased pulmonary arterial resistance might be associated with a lowered arterial oxygen saturation.

Mr Brock favoured the term persistent rather than patent ductus arteriosus. He thought that pulmonary hypertension was not uncommon in the

---

[*] Published in the *BHJ*.[86]

condition and that it falls after operation. He related the relative pulmonary stenosis in these cases to the persistence of the systolic murmur after closure of a ductus.

Dr Baker thought there was an unnatural selection in the cases of which Dr Shephard had spoken, and that pulmonary hypertension was found in older patients with P.D.A. Dr Holling questioned whether a lowered arterial saturation was reliable evidence of deficient pulmonary function in cases with septal defects in view of possible right to left shunts. Dr Shephard gave an assurance that error from this source had been guarded against. Mr Milstein asked whether organic changes were seen in the vessels of older patients. Dr Enticknap said the accounts in the literature were unsatisfactory but organic changes were not marked in patients with congenital heart disease. Mr Hill thought the cases of whom Dr Shephard had spoken were so highly selected that generalisations could not be made from them, and questioned whether it was correct to regard the left atrial pressure as always low in calculating the pulmonary vascular resistance. Dr Shephard agreed that the pulmonary capillary pressure would be better to take as the downstream pressure level in the pulmonary circuit but that this measurement had not been made in most of these cases. Dr Venner said that at least one of the cases of P.D.A. had had a high left atrial pressure at operation.

Dr Venner then spoke on the diastolic pressure gradient over the mitral valve.* He described the method by which these measurements had been made, and how continuous care had to be taken to eliminate artefacts. In several records he showed that in a mild case the pressure gradient was small, and large in a severe case. He compared a case in normal rhythm with one in auricular fibrillation to show how important atrial systole was in left ventricular filling if mitral stenosis was present. He showed that after mitral valvotomy there was no marked difference in diastolic filling time, also that after valvotomy the pressure pulse due to atrial systole was smaller indicating that the atrium was less tense. The pulse due to atrial systole seldom shows in the ventricle though in a long diastole the pressure in the two may approximate.

---

* Work published in the *BHJ*.[100;101]

The Heart Club

Dr Holling spoke of the marked fall in left ventricular pressure during the left ventricular relaxation which suggested that the left ventricle in effect sucked blood into it during early diastole. Dr Venner was doubtful whether this was the true interpretation of the findings and thought that the cause of the marked fall in pressure might be the pressure drop which is known to occur distal to a constriction.

Mr Brock agreed that it would be instructive to measure intracardiac pressure during a cardiac cycle when the mitral opening was occluded by the surgeons finger. Mr Hill said that Dr Venners remarks had shown him the importance of left ventricular pressure measurements.

The meeting closed at 10.30 pm.

Maurice Campbell
May 3rd 1954

May 1954

At the meeting in the Staff Common Room on Monday, May 3rd, there were present 16 members and by invitation Dr M. Sokolow of Los Angeles and Mr Jewsbury of Manchester.

The date and subject of the next meeting were not decided.

Mr Brock opened his talk on aortic stenosis with a radiograph illustrating his first sortie on the valve in 1947.* This was a retrograde aortic approach but now he believes a cardiac approach and the use of an expanding dilator to be preferable.

The measurement of pressure gradient over the valve may be the best method of assessing the severity of the stenosis. He had operated on 26 cases, 9 of which had an additional mitral lesion. 8 cases had died, two before any incision had been made. The criteria for selection of cases was still not worked out and Mr Brock pointed out that many of these cases were advanced cases with much calcification.

Dr Campbell voiced the meetings appreciation of the talk. He said it was clinical experience that patients with aortic stenosis do not, as a rule, deteriorate rapidly. Syncopal attacks appear to be an indication for surgery.

Dr Sokolow pointed out that whereas the right ventricle might stand up to a pressure three times its normal, the left ventricle failed under pressures about twice its normal. Was it therefore fair to say that the right ventricle stands strains less well than the right? He suggested that a mitral lesion may protect the left ventricle from the effects of an aortic lesion. Dr Holling asked for an explanation of how this could be, but no explanation could be given.

---

* Brock published on this problem in the *BMJ* in what he called a surgical essay.[102] The repetition of right and right is in the original minute. As the minutes state no explanation could be given and that remains the case on editing although the repetition of right suggests an error in the record. TT

The Heart Club

Dr Venner spoke of the relation between pressure gradient and blood flow through a valve.

The meeting closed at 10.20 pm.

Dec 3rd 1954
Maurice Campbell

December 1954

Twelve members were present at a meeting held in the Gordon Museum and the Staff Common Room on Friday, the 3rd December, 1954.

January 11th was suggested as the date of the next meeting when Dr Charles Baker will talk on the late results of Mitral Valvotomy.

Pathological specimens were shown.

Dr Campbell spoke of the inadequacies of the arrangements at Washington and the value of Lingua Franca as an international language. The development of visual aids to teaching had been highly developed. There was a craze for low fat diets for all people as a preventative of coronary disease, though the importance of fat as a predisposing cause was far from proven.

The surgery of A.S.D. and V.S.D. was being increasingly pursued and the use of crossed circulation from a suitable donor appeared hopeful, though in this procedure 3 of 9 donors had been seriously affected. The repair of a patent ostium primum* was difficult and efforts were being made to diagnose it before operation.

Ballistocardiography seemed valuable as a means of investigating the performance of the heart.

Sir Russell Brock spoke on various topics in connection with his visit to the International Cardiological Congress, Washington, 1954.

The question of direct and indirect operations for the relief of pulmonary stenosis was considered. It had been said that the direct operation was dangerous, attended with a high mortality and gave bad results. Some 2750 indirect operations had been done but only 180 direct ones. In most centres only one or two direct operations had been done, and it was not appreciated that the development of surgery of the open heart made the direct operation even more valuable. At Johns Hopkins Taussig had followed up the late results of 255, i.e. about half the cases of Fallots Tetralogy treated by the indirect operation. Good results had been obtained in 31% of cases operated

---

* See Glossary for ostium primum and secundum.

The Heart Club

on between the ages of 7 and 10 years, 62% between 2 and 8 years, and 62% between 12 and 20.[59]

The surgery of coronary thrombosis* was disappointing. Beck had now given up his anastomosis of aorta and coronary sinus. No satisfactory operation for mitral incompetence had yet been devised. The treatment of aortic incompetence devised by Hufnagel which consists of the insertion of a non-return valve in the descending aorta was dangerous and was not the answer.

Comparatively little fundamental work had been done with hypothermia and the performance of the artificial heart was unsatisfactory. In the treatment of A.S.D. the operation devised by Bjorck [sic] of splitting between the atria appears most hopeful. Attention had been paid to the diagnosis of the patent ostium primum because such cases were proving inoperable. The 16 cases of A.S.D. which had been operated on by Swan in Denver were early ones and had given good results.

Lillyhigh [sic] had used cross circulation from a donor with impressive results.

The meeting closed at 10.45 pm.

Jan 11th 1955
Maurice Campbell

---

* See coronary thrombosis in the glossary.
 This must be Viking Olov Björk. See Biographical Notes List 2.
 Clarence Walton Lillehei. See Biographical Notes List 2.

Tom Treasure

BRITISH MEDICAL JOURNAL
LONDON SATURDAY JULY 17 1954

RESULTS OF PULMONARY VALVOTOMY AND INFUNDIBULAR RESECTION IN 100 CASES OF FALLOT'S TETRALOGY

BY

MAURICE CAMPBELL, D.M., F.R.C.P.

D. C. DEUCHAR, M.D., M.R.C.P.

AND

Sir RUSSELL BROCK, M.S., F.R.C.S.

From the Cardiac Department and the Thoracic Surgical Unit, Guy's Hospital

We recently reported the results of Blalock–Taussig operations in 200 patients with morbus caeruleus, 165 of whom had Fallot's tetralogy (Campbell and Deuchar, 1953). We wish to add a parallel series of 100 patients operated on by Brock's direct methods, and a more detailed follow-up and analysis of the 61 operated on at Guy's Hospital up to the end of 1952 ; 12 others have been operated on at Guy's Hospital during 1953, and the remaining 27 at the Brompton Hospital either for or in conjunction with Dr. Paul Wood. The first attempts at direct relief of pulmonary stenosis by valvotomy were reported by Brock (1948) and by Brock and Campbell (1950a), the latter paper including an account of 15 patients in whom the valvular stenosis was part of Fallot's tetralogy. Infundibular resections were first reported by Brock (1949) and by Brock and Campbell (1950b), who described the results obtained in 11 patients.

Our purpose is to report the subsequent progress of these early patients and the results in those who have been operated on since. Valvotomy only was carried out in 37, infundibular resection only in 45, and a combined operation in 18 in which the stenosis was valvular and infundibular: sometimes these have been grouped with those who had valvotomy as there were too few for separate analysis. All these patients were thought to have Fallot's tetralogy. Two (Cases V65 and 26*) had already had a Blalock operation which had resulted in only moderate improvement.

The 61 patients who had been operated on at Guy's Hospital up to the end of 1952, when the details of the follow-up were arranged, are the only ones included in the full analysis. In 23 the operation was valvotomy, in 25 infundibular resection, and in the other 13 a combined operation.

Age and Sex.—Most of the patients were children. Their age distribution is shown in Table I. Only two were under 5 years of age, nearly a third were between 5 and 9, and nearly a third were between 10 and 15. The youngest was 4 and the oldest 34. Boys and men slightly predominated—33 against 28 girls and women. These figures are very similar to those for the patients who had subclavian–pulmonary anastomosis, but the former were a little older, because preference was being given to those who were older at the time these direct operations were started.

---

*Case numbers starting with V indicate those who had valvotomy, and the numbers without a prefix those who had infundibular resection only.

Disability.—This was graded (Campbell, 1948) as IV in 13, III in 28, II in 16, and I in 4 before operation. The disability was on the average a little less than in those who had anastomotic operations. This was because the anastomotic operations started in 1947 and the present ones in 1948, and the most disabled had generally

TABLE I.—*Age Distribution of Patients and Deaths after Operation*

	No. of Cases in Each Age Group					
Age in years:	0–4	5–9	10–14	15–19	20 +	Total
Pulmonary valvotomy alone and combined	2	12	9	7	6	36
Infundibular resection	0	7	10	3	5	25
Both operations	2	19	19	10	11	61
Deaths after operation	0	3	2	2	4	11
Proportion of deaths	14%		11%	20%	36%	18%
Proportion of good results	52%		84%	60%	54%	64%

been chosen for operation first. The fact that the patients were older and had survived to this age implies that they had not always been the most severe cases or they would have died sooner, but the older patients chosen for operation were generally losing ground, and sometimes seriously so. We think that the slighter disability and the greater age (with its greater operative risk) balance each other and make the two groups closely comparable. The disability grading in the valvotomy series differs from that in the resection series only by including more patients in grade IV and fewer in grade II.

Cardiac Catheterization in Diagnosis

The general findings of catheterization and the value of various special investigations in the diagnosis of morbus caeruleus, and their limitations in the assessment of the results of anastomotic operations, have been discussed (Campbell and Deuchar, 1953). Catheterization has a more valuable place in assessing the haemodynamic changes after direct operations (see later), and has the same value in diagnosis and an added value in elucidating the anatomy of the right ventricular outflow tract, for its precise anatomy is more important to the surgeon than before an anastomotic operation.

Physical signs may be helpful but are not reliable in differentiating valvular and infundibular stenosis. A good angiocardiogram may demonstrate clearly the exact site of the stenosis present in Fallot's tetralogy, but often it does not give a decisive answer or may even lead to a

4880

The question of direct or indirect (that is Blalocks) operation for the relief of pulmonary stenosis was discussed again in the meeting in December 1954. Brock and Campbell had considered the matter at length in a paper in the British Heart Journal 1950[59] and reported their results with direct operations here in the British Medical Journal in 1954[27]. Brocks view, as stated in the minutes for December 1954 was that it was not appreciated that the development of surgery of the open heart made the direct operation even more valuable.

165

PULMONARY VALVOTOMY 9

In this way the site of the obstruction is confirmed, any other abnormality such as an infundibular stenosis is discovered, and a measure is established to compare with the pressures after valvotomy (Figure 5).

A special curved probe, 4 mm. in diameter (Figure 6) is now passed to confirm the presence of the valvular obstruction and to

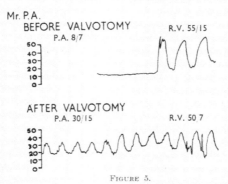

FIGURE 5.
Electromanometric pressure tracings during pulmonary valvotomy. After valvotomy the pressures in pulmonary artery and right ventricle are approximated, and there is a good pulse wave in the artery.

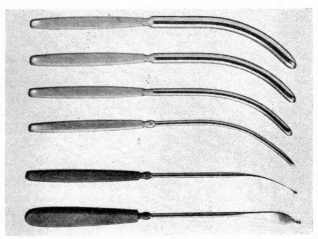

FIGURE 6.
From above downwards: dilators, 1·25 cm., 1·0 cm., 0·7 cm., and 0·4 cm. in diameter, and a valvotome in profile and from the front.

Brock had modified a range of instruments to dilate and to cut a stenosed pulmonary valve.[250]

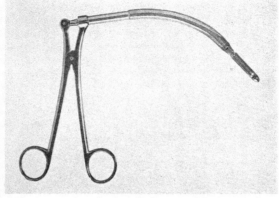

FIGURE 7.
Two-bladed expanding dilator.

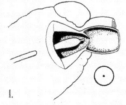
1.

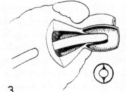
3.

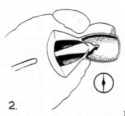
2.

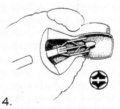
4.

FIGURE 8.
1. The valvotome approaching the stenosed valve. 2. The stenosis has been divided and the valvotome tip now lies in the pulmonary artery. 3. The orifice is enlarged with a dilator. 4. The expanding dilator is opened in the valve orifice, splitting it widely.

Brock a dilator for the pulmonary valve.[250]

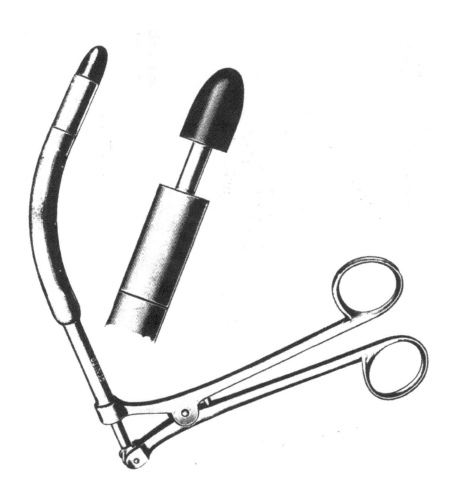

Brocks infundibular punch was designed to cut and retain obstructing muscle from within the beating right ventricle.

January 1955
Eleven members were present at a meeting of the Peacock Club in the Wardens House on January 11th.

The date of the next meeting was fixed for February 22nd, 1955, the subject of discussion to be 1) Coarctation of the Aorta, and 2) Atrial Septal Defect, the opening speakers to be Dr Campbell and Dr Baylis.

Dr Baker spoke on the late results of mitral valvotomy. Of 45 patients with a good result from operation 6 deteriorated in the second year, 11 in the 3rd year; but of 21 excellent results 15 had remained in good health over 4 years.[*]

Prognosis depends primarily on what the surgeon is able to do at operation; on the whole patients with pulmonary hypertension respond better, neither minor degrees of rheumatic activity nor mitral regurgitation appear to affect the result. There is little evidence of re-stenosis but deterioration, if it occurs, happens quietly and is probably due to myocardial degeneration, for atrial fibrillation often occurs. In the decision whether to operate or not the opinion of the patient whether he is losing ground or not is important, and surgical skill is an important factor to be considered in prognosis.

Sir Russell Brock: The functional state of the valve matters more than the size of the orifice when considering prognosis.

Four types of valve may be described:

1. Valve of small central lumen, pliable, not calcified.
2. Fibrous valve.
3. One commissure calcified. Chordae tendineae fused and regurgitation free.
4. Valve solid with calcification.

At the end of operation these may be.

1. A normal valve.
2. Only one commissure open.

---

[*] This study of 45 longer follow-up patients was published in the *BMJ*.[103]

The Heart Club

3. Only a central hole.
4. Fibro calcareous valve.

Dr Campbell believed relapse was due to myocardial degeneration; usually a good mechanical result at operation is followed by a good clinical result.

Mr Ian Hill: There is a greater danger of causing incompetence when operating on a mild case. Operation diminished risk of emboli. The gross bronchitic does not do well after operation. There is no doubt the surgeon improves with practice so that mitral valvotomy should remain in specialist hands.

Dr Baker: In prognosis the age of the disease is of more importance than the age of the patient.

Feb 22nd 1955
Maurice Campbell

Present author's commentary:
In the meeting in January 1955 Charles Baker and Russell Brock set out what the Club had learned from their first-hand experience of operations for mitral stenosis and its outcomes which they reported in their series of BMJ papers.[63;103;118]

The attitude to operation for mitral stenosis in the post war years is described in the introduction: Peace returns to Guys Hospital 1945-1948. The received wisdom of the was expounded by James McKenzie[40-43;45] and Thomas Lewis.[47] The myocardium was regarded as the primary cause of the patients trouble, not the valve. But we know that from the formation of the Peacock Club, Brock had valvotomy in mind. He had written in the *BMJ* in 1948:

> When one examines the heart post mortem in patients dying of valvular disease and contemplates the minute size of the orifice through which the whole lifeblood of the body has to be forced it is impossible not to feel that this simple mechanical obstruction must be capable of relief by surgery.[30]

At the time he was writing his paper about relieving pulmonary stenosis[30] by operation in the context of congenital heart disease, but aware of Souttars case in 1925, we know that he also had mitral stenosis in mind.[36] The first successful operations for mitral stenosis in the post war era were by Charles Bailey, Dwight Harken and Russell Brock, all in 1948.[48;49;63] It was soon evident that the physical opening of the valve aperture reversed much or all of the symptoms, depending primarily on what the surgeon is able to do at operation as Charles Baker said in the *January 1955* meeting of the Club.

In the previous year in March 1954, Paul Wood had delivered the Strickland Goodall lecture An appreciation of mitral stenosis.[328;329] According to Sir John McMichael, Wood concluded his lecture with the words The trouble with mitral stenosis – is mitral stenosis reversing the doctrine of the Mackenzie Lewis era.[45]

In the following table (P.172) the changing attitudes to surgical operation for mitral stenosis can be followed. In successive editions of Prices Textbook of Medicine[330] mitral stenosis was seen as possibly amenable to surgery, then contra-indicated but by 1956 mitral valvotomy was standard treatment.

The Heart Club

Frederick Price was Consulting Physician to the National Hospital for Diseases of the Heart. The successive editions of his textbook from 1922 to 1956 track the changes in received opinion on the question of operating to relieve mitral stenosis.[330]

Date	A Text Book of the Practice of Medicine. Frederick W Price
1922	No mention of surgery.
1926	No mention of surgery.
1929	Nearly a page long entry citing Samways, Lauder Brunton 1902, Doyen, Cutler and Levine 1923, the experimental work of Strickland Goodall and Rogers 1924, and Souttar 1925.
1933	A page long entry almost identical to 1929 but he adds a reference to Cushing.
1937	The long account was omitted and replace with: Surgical treatment in the form of valvulotomy, both by the auricular and ventricular routes, has been performed in a number of cases of mitral stenosis. This procedure should be regarded as in an experimental stage.
1941	The same with the addition of The mortality is high. Again, the change from mitral stenosis to incompetence is of doubtful value.
1946	Surgical treatment in the form of valvulotomy, both by the auricular and ventricular routes, has been performed in a number of cases of mitral stenosis with the object of enlarging the orifice. This procedure is contra-indicated. The mortality is high. Again, the change from mitral stenosis to incompetence is of doubtful value.
1950	Surgical treatment has been performed in a number of cases of mitral stenosis. In the earlier ones the procedure consisted in stretching the orifice by the fingers. Later a valvulotome has been employed with the object of converting the stenosed valve into an incompetent one. In the case of both the mortality is high, and in the latter the change from stenosis to incompetence is of doubtful value. Both procedures are contra-indicated.
1956	Price had retired from editing the book aged over 80 and the section on valvular heart disease was by Wallace Brigden. It is over two pages long and starts Mitral valvotomy is indicated in all patients in whom serious obstruction to the flow of blood through the stenosed valve is the dominant functional disorder and ends saying that in three quarters of patients the results are good or excellent.

February 1955
At a meeting of the Peacock Club on Tuesday, February 22nd, 1955, there were present 14 members. Pathological specimens were shown in the Gordon Museum and the meeting then adjourned to the Wardens House.

It was suggested that the next meeting would be on May 3rd, when Sir Russell Brock would talk about the Detroit Conference. It was decided that Dr Neil, Dr Dow and Dr Rheinhoff* should be invited to become members of the Club.

Dr Campbell opened the discussion on Coarctation of the Aorta. The seriousness of the condition is indicated by the finding that 70% of patients are less than 20 years old and only 10% over 30. Coarctation is seldom associated with other congenital abnormalities. Heart failure is the commonest mode of death but cerebral haemorrhage and rupture of the aorta also occur. Operative mortality, except in complicated cases, is not high. The indications for operation are not yet firmly established. To decide prognosis after operation will require a long term follow-up.

Dr Bayliss [sic] stressed the importance of changes in the medial coat of the aorta. It is still undecided whether hypertension or congenital aneurysms at the base of the brain are more important in the causation of cerebral haemorrhage. Examples of Turners syndrome with coarctation prove on skin biopsy to be males.

Sir Russell Brocks opinion was that coarctation should always be corrected surgically unless there are good reasons against doing this. The object of the operation is to prevent progressive hypertension and this has been done in all but one of 52 patients. In this series there were 6 deaths closely connected with operation, the first death being the 24th case operated on. In most big series of cases the operative mortality was about 6%. His own opinion was that aortic grafting should only be done when absolutely necessary but he had had to do it in 15 of 42 cases. Constriction of the aorta is not

---

* This is probably Dr W. F. Rienhoff of Johns Hopkins who had been an exchange visitor a few years earlier.
 This is likely to be John Baylis. He wrote in *BHJ* with Campbell on coarctation.[104]
See Biographical Notes List 1.

The Heart Club

the only fault in coarctation, for the aorta is also hypoplastic. The distinction between adult and infantile coarctation is a very fine one. He had not noticed aortic valve disease in any of the patients on whom he had operated.

Hypotension is a great help in operative technique but after operation reactive hypertension may often be troublesome. The etiology of this condition is not known.

Operation should be done at as early an age as possible and Crafoord had shown that the anastomosis will grow with the child.

Dr Baker asked about the danger of bacterial endocarditis after operation.

Mr Ian Hill agreed with the value of controlled hypotension at operation and the advisability of operation at an early age. No restriction of activity was necessary afterwards.

In answer to a question of Dr Suzman, Dr Baylis replied that of 22 patients with aortic diastolic murmurs only 4 had a wide pulse pressure.

The general opinion was in favour of operation before puberty.

The meeting adjourned at 11.20 pm.

March 29th 1955
Maurice Campbell

Tom Treasure

March 1955

At a meeting of the club on March 29th 1955, Sir Russell Brock described recent developments in cardiac surgery in the U.S.A.

During the previous six months the direct operation on the stenosed pulmonary valve had become the method of choice; the trans-arterial route was being tried but with indifferent success.

Lillehei in Minneapolis attempts to repair ventricular septal defects only if there is evidence of progressive pulmonary hypertension. He has also devised a method of dealing with transposition of the great vessels. Atrial septal defect and its repair has been attracting great interest. Much has been written about the distinction of ostium primum from ostium secundum defects. The former carries a high risk at operation.

Lillehei has used cross circulation in 31 patients with ventricular septal defect and 5 with Fallots Tetralogy. The amount of cross circulation required is measured in terms of the flow through the azygous vein which can be calculated from body size; twice the azygous factor is usually employed. Various technical defects have played a large part in the high mortality due to the procedure. The operation takes around 2½ hours, the cross circulation being maintained for about ½ hour. The method is regarded as being a temporary expedient. Experiments have been made using the dogs lung as an aerator.

Dr Harken and Dr Bayley* continue to devise unsatisfactory operations for mitral regurgitation. Bayley has used the aortic route for aortic stenosis. Hufnagel has had a high mortality with his artificial valves in cases of aortic regurgitation, but has dealt only with advanced cases.

The Gibbon heart lung machine is expensive and complicated. In arterial reconstructions artificial materials are being increasingly used.

Dec 18th 1955
Maurice Campbell

---

* Almost certainly Charles Bailey given the context. Biographical Notes List 2
See Gibbon heart lung machine in the Glossary and Gibbon Biographical Notes List 2.
Signature on the minute doesnt match the date of the next meeting.

The Heart Club

December 1955

Seventeen members were present at a meeting held on December 15th 1955. Pathological specimens were shown in the Gordon Museum.

The proposed date of the next meeting was January 17th 1956, the subject to be Atrial Septal Defect. This was later changed to January 30th, the subject to be Ventricular Defect.

Dr Campbell opened a discussion on the surgical treatment of aortic stenosis. Five of the 16 patients operated on at Guys up to December, 1954 had derived considerable benefit. For a physician the difficulty was to select, before the valve became inoperable, the cases who were going to deteriorate.

Sir Russell Brock pointed out that the operative mortality has lessened in the last year to 6 deaths in 50 cases. Congenital aortic stenosis in young people offered the best chance of success. Judging by the cases presented to him deterioration in aortic stenosis might take place at any age. The height of the left ventricular pressure might indicate which cases were going to deteriorate. Causes of failure are calcification of the valve, failure of the myocardium, and the danger of producing aortic regurgitation.[*]

Dr Charles Baker said how slight the first signs of a rapid deterioration might be, but that operation could not be freely advised until the operative mortality was low, say less than 2.

Dr Suzman thought that angina and the occurrence of left ventricular strain pattern in the E.C.G. might be indication for operation.

Mr Ross described the technique of left atrial puncture and the insertion of a catheter to measure the left ventricular pressure. In 14 cases there had been one death due to haematoma of the lung two weeks after catheterisation, 1 pneumothorax, 1 pulmonary oedema, and 1 temporary heart block.

Dr Fleming gave reasons why measurements of the pressure gradient across the aortic valve at operation were best done with a catheter in the left ventricular outflow track and a needle in the aorta. After a successful operation

---

[*] This was a continuing challenge for Brock, later described in the *BMJ*. [102]

there is a reduction in the mean systolic pressure gradient and a shortening of the time of the upstroke of the aortic pressure tracing.

In aortic stenosis a reduced and fixed cardiac output leads to syncope; left ventricular failure, to breathlessness, and angina disproportion between coronary flow and left ventricular work. E.C.G. changes were helpful; phonocardiography, ballistocardiography and dye dilution curves might be helpful.

Dr Reinhold described characteristics phonocardiographic changes in aortic stenosis. The first sound is accentuated and split, the aortic second sound may be accentuated, and because of the delay of aortic closure there is no splitting of the second sound in the pulmonary area.

Mr Milsteins technique of left atrial puncture differed from that of Mr Ross in that his needle took a more oblique route and passed through the lung. This disadvantage was offset by a greater likelihood of reaching the left atrium.*

Jan 30th 1956
Maurice Campbell

---

* Brock, Milstein and Ross wrote on both left atrial and left ventricular punctures in *Thorax* 1956. [105]

The Heart Club

January 1956

Twenty one members were present at a meeting on January 30th, 1956, in the Wardens House.

The date of the next meeting was fixed for March 12th, the subject for discussion to be Atrial Septal Defect on which Dr Catherine Neal and Dr Suzman would speak.

Dr Campbell opened the discussion on ventricular septal defect.* This lesion occurs in about 30% of cases of congenital heart disease either in isolation or combined with other defects. No significant progress was made in our knowledge of the conditions until cardiac catheterisation was introduced. V.S.D. may be divided according to the size of the defect and in the most severe cases by the pulmonary hypertension and reversal of shunt. The major dividing line of mild into severe cases occurs when the defect is 1 cm. wide when the pulmonary flow approaches 15 litres. V.S.D. may be distinguished from A.S.D. for the pulmonary second sound is less commonly split; on x-ray the right ventricle is enlarged in both conditions but only in V.S.D. is the left ventricle also enlarged. The electrocardiogram may show right ventricular preponderance in A.S.D. and preponderance of either ventricle in V.S.D. Incomplete right bundle branch block is also less commonly encountered in V.S.D. Pulmonary hypertension and shunt reversal occurs late in A.S.D. and earlier, at 10 to 20 years, in V.S.D.

V.S.D. may be associated with pulmonary stenosis and in other cases an aortic cusp is involved in the lesion giving rise to aortic incompetence. The importance of overriding aorta has been unjustly emphasised and such a condition cannot be diagnosed before the P.M. room. No reason for retaining the diagnosis of Eisenmengers Complex can be given.

Dr Brotmacher regarded diagnosis from the catheter findings as a matter of assessing probabilities. If the ventricular sample contains 1 volume more oxygen per cent than the atrial a V.S.D. is likely. Many samples must be taken to recognise the effect of blood streaming. In A.S.D. right ventricular

---

* This is an example of Campbells planned documentation of natural history of congenital conditions. He published twice in the *BHJ* on VSD.[106;107]
Leon Brotmacher was the first author on the subsequent publication.[106]

pressure in late stages may greatly exceed the left. This seldom happens with V.S.D. and a P.A.P. of 50mm is likely to have a bad prognosis.

Measurement of the circulation times from heart cavities may aid diagnosis. Selective angiocardiography may also help. After operation all evidence of the lesion may disappear.

Dr Reinhold said that in A.S.D. the venous pulse may show a characteristic pattern which perhaps is not found in V.S.D. V.S.D. is the fourth most common cause of death by cardiac failure in infants; A.S.D. is the commonest.

Sir Russell Brock asked that the natural history of the condition should be studied with particular attention to the condition in infants. Surgically it is important to distinguish a common atrio-ventricular canal. The concept of overriding aorta (Eisenmengers Syndrome) is confusing mumbo jumbo.

If a malformation gives rise to a small systemic circulation difficulties occur at operation, so a Fallots is easier to deal with than an uncomplicated V.S.D. Also the isolated lesion may involved the A V valve mechanism.

Hypothermia is particularly dangerous if the ventricular muscle is in poor condition.

March 12th 1956
Maurice Campbell

The Heart Club

March 1956

A meeting of the Peacock Club was held on March 12th, 1956 at 8 p.m.

Dr Catherine Neill opened the discussion on Atrial Septal Defect.[*] In infancy a pointer towards the diagnosis is a discrepancy between the forcible precordial beat and the feeble peripheral pulse. The exact diagnosis of the condition, however, is difficult in the first two years of life and again when the shunt has been reversed. A large V wave in the jugular pulse is suggestive. Often a loud systolic murmur is heard in the pulmonary area and this is well heard through to the back. The diagnosis is unlikely unless there is wide splitting of the 2nd sound. x-ray shows enlargement of the right atrium and pulmonary artery and the left atrium and ventricle should be small. There is no certain way to distinguish Ostium Primum lesions from Ostium Secundum. Early cardiac failure is in favour of ostium primum. A pan systolic murmur, enlargement of the left ventricle and left axis deviation suggest that mitral regurgitation is associated and make an ostium primum lesion more likely.

Dr Suzman described the E.C.G. features. Right bundle branch block commonly occurred and a notching of the primary R wave in the QRS complex should be looked for in unipolar leads.

Dr Campbell though he agreed with Dr Neills observations on the early onset of failure in ostium primum lesions, had observed that such a lesion was compatible with long survival. A.S.D. in general is less common in males and the sex preponderance increases with the age group of the patients, though the reason for this is not clear. Once symptoms occur the downhill course is rapid. The end stages are characterised either by cardiac failure or increasing cyanosis. If infancy is survived death occurs most frequently in the 4th decade. Anomalous pulmonary drainage appears to be less well tolerated than simple atrial septal defect.

---

[*] An example of Dr Campbells work to document the natural history of congenital disease. This was published soon after with Catherine Neil and Samuel Suzman in the *BMJ*.[108]

See glossary for precordial beat.

Dr Reinhold showed examples of the large V wave in A.S.D. and observed that the split in the 2nd sound is fixed in time.*

Sir Russell Brock described the considerable advances made in the surgical treatment of the lesion. In suitable cases the operation was now devoid of risk and the technique of hypothermia was now practical and satisfactory. The condition should be dealt with before the heart began to fail.

Dr Brotmacher dealt with the diagnosis of the lesion by cardiac catheterisation and stated that the catheter was more likely to go through the defect if the approach was made through the saphenous vein. The effect of temporary closure of the lesion might be observed by the use of a balloon ended catheter. Anomalous pulmonary drainage was particularly difficult to diagnose and Sir Russell thought that a diagnosis of the condition before operation could only be made with certainty if the pulmonary veins entered the superior vena cava.

Dr Fleming mentioned the use of dye dilution curves in diagnosis and described the condition in which pulmonary veins drained into the coronary sinus.

Dr Ashmore said that a possible technique in dealing with complete pulmonary venous drainage into a persistent left superior vena cava was to anastomose the superior vena cava to the left atrial appendage, but it was questionable whether the left superior vena cava should then be ligatured.

---

* This work was published subsequently in the *BHJ*.[109]
 The last meeting for which there is a record in the book of Minutes and it is unsigned. I think there may have been no more meetings in this format and the year is that of Dr Campbells retirement.

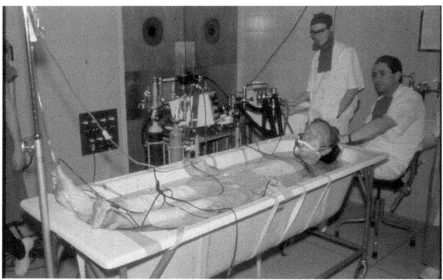

The natural history of atrial septal defect as was discussed in the final meeting of the Peacock Club in March 1956 and Brock commented that the defect could be closed with hypothermia. This was the method: surface cooling in a cold bath with added ice to a body temperature of about 30°C. The picture is from Alison Hill from her fathers collection. I am not sure where the picture was taken but the master of the technique at the time was Thomas Holmes Sellors at The Middlesex Hospital.[316]

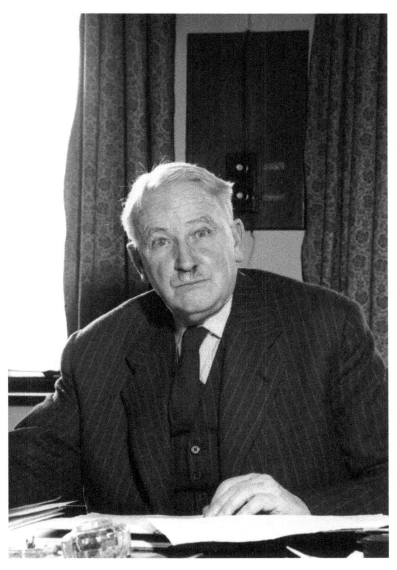

Maurice Campbell (1891–1973) photographed in 1956, the last year of the Club and the year of Dr Campbells retirement.

Three 'Blue Babies' –
their lives 1944–2017

Geraldine West, John Hunt and Xerxes Talati were born in 1944, 1948 and 1950 respectively. They were 'blue babies'; the underlying cause in all three was Fallot's Tetralology. The combination of obstruction of the blood flow to the lungs and a defect in the ventricular septum (commonly referred to as a 'hole in the heart') meant that their blood was never adequately oxygenated and remained a dark purple rather than the bright red of oxygenated blood. This gave their skin the blue tinge called cyanosis.

In his lecture to Guy's students in January 1946, Dr Maurice Campbell declined to say much about 'the grossly cyanosed cases for which not much in the way of treatment can be done beyond controlling the activities of the patient'.[17] Following the visit of Dr Alfred Blalock of Johns Hopkins Hospital in September 1947 Dr Campbell gave a very different lecture.[19] He was completely converted. The first three of his patients who had been operated on by Alfred Blalock had been brought back to see him, and he had received word about the others. In nine out of ten there was a dramatic improvement. He described one, who had rarely walked more than about 10 yards, 'running about all day: the parents say it is very difficult to stop him'. He admitted 'I was almost alarmed at the amount they were doing. I did not appreciate how much a child, suddenly relieved of his lifelong disability, might want to do.'[19] There had been a complete turnaround in his view about this disease and the possibility of surgery.

Dr Campbell knew that in the natural way of things, most blue babies had died young and the majority 'exist rather than live'.[19] But now word had gone out that these patients could be helped. By November 1948 Dr Campbell had seen 460 patients with congenital heart disease of whom were 340 cyanosed at rest. The first part of the patients' stories is during the era of the Peacock Club when these patients had 'palliative' operations for Fallot's Tetralogy, just improving to a degree the blood flow to their lungs. The second part of their stories covers the subsequent course of events up to the time of writing this book. They had further surgery to repair the structure of their hearts so as to restore, as far as possible, normal function. Their lives have been punctuated by complications and treatments but they remain alive and are well.

The Heart Club

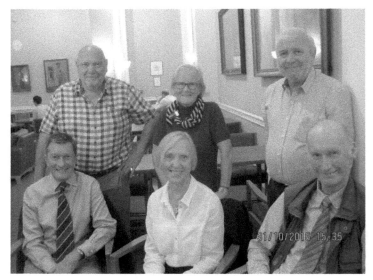

In the front row are Xerxes Talati, Geraldine West and John Hunt, born as Blue Babies. Behind are Christopher Lawrence (historian of medicine), Kate Bull (childrens heart specialist and author of Open Hearts) and Tom Treasure (heart surgeon). The photograph was taken in the Housman Room, the academic senior common room of University College London, in October 2016.

Geraldine West from her birth 1944 to surgical palliation in 1954

GW – I was born on 11th June 1944 with Fallots Tetralogy. My parents were told that there was nothing to be done and that my life expectancy was seven to fifteen years. The first of my nine lives was lost when I was just eleven days old. I was asleep in my cot when a bomb exploded near our home in South East London. A wardrobe door was blown across the cot, protecting me from the roof which fell on top of it. My grandfather dug me out, unscathed. We were rehoused in a Victorian terraced house in Woolwich, which my parents later bought at auction for £120.

I was my parents third child and by the time I was six, my mother had had two more children. Although I knew of course that I was not able to do the things my siblings could do, I never questioned this – it was just the way things were.

As I was not able to walk more than a few steps without needing to rest, my life was limited to our living room and my push-chair. I have no memory of playing with toys except Meccano, which I loved, or having any interaction with my siblings. I did a lot of drawing, cutting and pasting paper and generally making a mess on the table. My father called me Miss Snippets. From an early age, he took me to the library almost every week. I loved to read and read my way through Enid Blytons *Noddy* and *Faraway Tree* books, later graduating to *The Famous Five* and *The Secret Seven*. My parents were avid listeners to BBCs Home Service so the backdrop to my early years was *Woman's Hour, Mrs Dale's Diary, The Archers*, the radio plays which I loved and the news of course. My mother would leave me outside, in my pram and later in my pushchair, in the tiny area of paving that was our front garden, for me to get some fresh air. A memory of this was my mother rushing out of our front door to tell our neighbour that the King had died.* I was a much loved and nurtured and I believe a well-grounded and contented child from the start.

There was only one more terraced house between us and a church school. As I approached my fifth birthday, my parents application for me to go to this school was turned down on health grounds. I am told a long, hard-fought battle ensued before I was eventually allowed to attend. I remember my first day there very clearly, with the kindly, very thin, pale-skinned and extremely old (!) teacher, the dappled mare rocking horse, the Wendy house, the sand pit and so many toys.

The school was housed in a Victorian building with large rooms and very high ceilings. Fires in the classrooms were the only form of heating – I often felt cold at school. One incident I remember. To begin with a chair was provided for me at morning assemblies. However on this particular morning one of the teachers insisted that I should stand with the other children. After a while my heart began pounding in my chest – it felt as though the whole of my inside was jumping up and down. I came to in the school kitchen, with people peering down at me. I was not made to stand in assembly again! Unless the weather was fine and I could sit on a bench outside, I stayed in the classroom at playtimes. My mother took me home for lunch and would keep me at home if she felt I was too tired to go back to school for the afternoon session.

---

* George VI 1895–1952

Two things happened in these early years which transformed my life chances. The first was the NHS. We were not well off. We would in todays jargon be just about managing. We had enough for modest needs, for outings and holidays at the seaside, but my parents would not have been able to pay for the treatment I was to have. Then, when I was six, my mother was approached by someone in the street who told her that her cousin was one of the leading heart specialists at Guys and that she could arrange for me to see him. His name was Dr Campbell. I owe her my life and am eternally grateful to her.

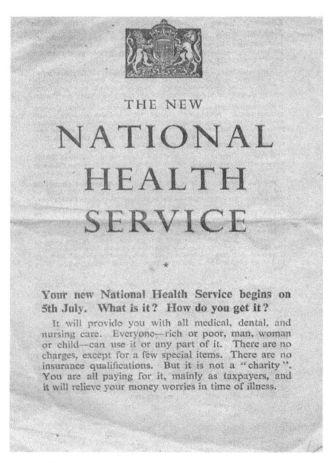

The flyer that was circulated to announce the National Health Service on 5th July 1948. Geraldine West and John Hunt give thanks for the NHS in their accounts.

Something else happened that has resonated throughout my life. It was a Sunday in the autumn of 1951 and I had that afternoon been admitted to Guys. My parents had gone home, there were no other children in the ward and feeling alone and frightened I hid under the bedclothes and cried. Some grown-ups came to my bedside and began talking about me and I heard one of them say She is very brave. I felt ashamed of myself – my parents had instilled in me the need to be brave. I determined then and there that I would be brave and would not cry again. It would be 13 years before I cried in hospital again. Being brave whatever happens, has enabled me, for the most part, to keep calm and carry on.

Early in 1952 I was admitted to hospital again, this time to The Middlesex, into the care of Thomas Holmes Sellors. I remember waiting with my parents in that magnificent entrance hall, being met by a nurse in a bright blue uniform with a white apron and hat, being taken up in the lift to the third floor and through the double doors to De Morgan ward. It had been agreed that Mr Holmes Sellors would operate. My parents told me in later years that the operation was experimental and had not been performed in this country before.* I am not sure if this was in fact the case or if so when they were told. However, it was not successful and I came close to becoming a statistic. My parents were called to the hospital late one night as it was thought that I might not survive til morning. I remember being in an oxygen tent with its cool, slightly sharp smelling air, a nurse sitting by my bedside at a small table with a lamp and a green baize cloth shielding the light and hands coming through the plastic from time to time to give me a drink or take my temperature. I have no memory of my parents being there.

On a cold dark night with snow on the ground I was wrapped in a blanket and taken with my parents in a taxi to a convalescent home at West Wickham in Kent. This home was being run, according to my mother, by a member of the Gestapo. I was very unhappy there. The childrens beds, in a long room, faced either the walls on either side or, in my case, floor to ceiling windows looking out onto trees and shrubs. I was not a nervous child but I remember watching carefully at night to see whether large animals or other creatures were lurking in the shrubbery. I do not know how

---

* We have so far failed to establish exactly what was attempted and in what sense it was experimental. TT&GW

unwell I was, but in the two weeks I was there, I was not allowed out of bed, except for the bed to be made. The beds were partially screened so I could not see the other children and no toys were provided. My parents were only allowed to visit once a week and the childrens letters home were – astonishingly – dictated by Matron. Although my mother was anxious about removing me from medical care, we agreed a code – if I was so unhappy that I wanted to come home I was to put three kisses at the end of my next letter, which I did. My parents complained to The Middlesex about the way this home was being run.

As a result of this operation I was less well than previously. I would be ten before I was well enough to go back to school. After a while a home tutor called Miss Fisk came to the house two mornings a week.

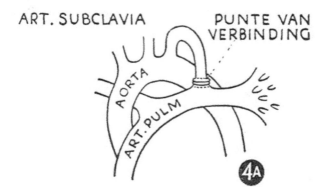

A drawing of the subclavian to pulmonary artery anastomosis devised in a collaboration between the paediatrician Helen Taussig, the laboratory technician Vivien Thomas and the surgeon Alfred Blalock.[18] Geraldine West had this operation performed by Thomas Holmes Sellors in 1954. This drawing comes from a paper published in Cape Town in 1954 by Michael Jordaan who trained with Brock and attended the Peacock Club in 1949 and 1950 before returning to South Africa.[236]

In 1954 I was admitted to The Middlesex for a second operation – this time the Blalock. I remember my father visiting me the day before and saying that after this I would be able to run around like other children. And this was indeed the case – to quote Dr Jane Somerville – this blue child became pink. I was well.

Everyone made such a fuss of me in hospital that I never minded being there, I always felt cared for and safe and – I suppose – a bit special. Being thrown out of the nest at such an early age made me more outgoing and confident than I might otherwise have been and taught me how to be at ease with adults. The only sadness was waving goodbye to my parents at the end of visiting times. I could see the whole length of Berners Street from the windows of De Morgan ward. I would wave to them and they would wave back until they were out of sight. That Christmas my parents bought me, against their better judgement, longed-for roller skates. On Christmas morning skating outside the house, I fell heavily and had my first migraine.

John Hunt from his birth in 1948 and early life up to surgical palliation in 1954

JH – I was born in August 1948 (the year the NHS was founded!), a Blue Baby with Fallots Tetralogy and according to the report I have by Sir Russell Brock (subsequently Lord Brock), at the age of five I could only walk about 50 yards before getting breathless and would constantly squat. In the same report Dr Paul Wood interpreted the findings as suggesting Fallots Tetralogy with a bidirectional shunt. On my sixth birthday on 25th August 1954 Sir Russell carried out the Brock Procedure, as the hole-in-heart surgery could not be carried out in those early days.

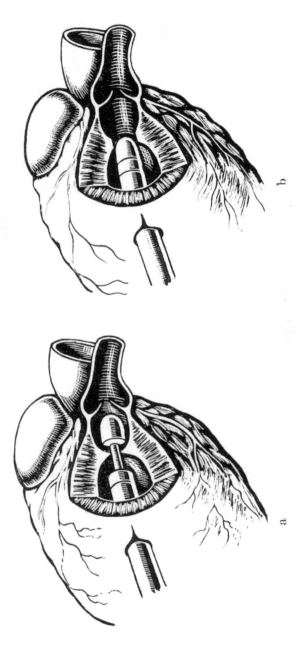

The punch devised by Russell Brock to allow a direct operation on the obstruction caused by the muscle in the right ventricle below the pulmonary valve.[27;59]

Tom Treasure

Being born in the middle of a family of nine children in a rural Northamptonshire cottage I suppose it was only natural I should find independence was a useful asset to have. I remember my many early train journeys to hospital in London with a mixture of memories. On the one hand I have pictures of looking at steam trains out of the windows on the journey to London but always mixed with an element of fear over what I might have to go through in hospital. In those days injections, removing stitches and drainage pipes, cameras to the heart via the nose and the various necessary procedures are all pictures which represent those early fears and have remained with me but happily in hindsight, all are seen as positive things to get me where I am now. I think my most happy memory after coming home from hospital and two weeks in Maids Morton Convalescent home when I was six, was the sight of my birthday present waiting in our front room with the sun shining on my new model farm!

My independence stood me in good stead in that during the almost five months away from home, I had relatively few visits, with mother looking after the large family and father working hard but I was quite happy with the friends I had made in hospital. I remember one particularly outstanding German nurse we called Sooty, who was quite strict but such a caring and fun loving lady that she still stands out in my mind from those early days. I often wonder what happened to her.

It might be worth mentioning how my siblings treated the slightly unusual circumstances around their brother. The five younger siblings were either not born or were very young when I had my operations and remember little or nothing about them. The eldest brother died some years ago and he had left home early so I did not have much contact with him. However I have spoken to my elder brother and sister who are only four and five years respectively older than I am and learnt a few stories from them. I never thought of either of them as being religious but found it interesting that my sister recalls saying prayers for me during the crisis times and my brother tells me that he remembers, at the age ten, on the day of my first operation in 1954, standing looking at the night sky and saying a prayer for my survival. He says that he saw a dazzling light in the sky and took that as a sign I would be alright! My brother would carry me on his shoulders on some of his walks when I would be puffed and blue and what now seems to be a short walk for me (I have moved back to where I was born) seemed a long adventure in those days. He tells me that he remembers the incredible devotion and resolve of my mother towards me and although I know my father was not so available, I was always conscious of the fact that he worked very hard in keeping a good house and large family in order. Big sister visited me in hospital on occasions and recalls that as we had no telephone, there were urgent calls to the local butcher from the hospital to get them to pass on messages that I was perhaps in a dangerous state and asking the parents to go to the hospital. She also reminded me that I used to have regular visits from a priest in the Brompton Oratory who became a good friend in my early days but I cant remember his name.

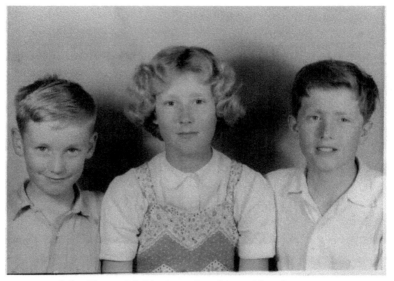

John Hunt with his sister Cynthia and brother Peter.

That first operation, a Brock procedure, was at Brompton Hospital in 1954 and successfully improved the blood flow to John Hunt's lungs, making him less blue and improving his exercise tolerance greatly.

Xerxes Talati from birth in 1950 to surgical palliation in 1954

Zarine, Xerxes' mother talked with us in December 2016. The family lived in Zanzibar. She recalled Xerxes' early childhood. He was blue from birth and would become distressed with feeding. He learned to stand and walk but even a few steps would exhaust him. He would squat down and sometimes fainted.

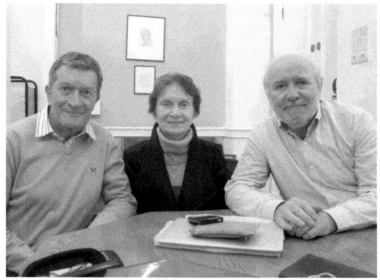

Xerxes Talati, his mother Zarine and Tom Treasure in the Housman Room at University College London in 2017.

Xerxes picked up the story – I was born in March 1950 and it was my maternal grandfather who noticed the blueish complexion. As luck would have it, he had qualified at Guys Hospital at about the same time as Brock. Grandfather then wrote a letter to Brock explaining about me. I remember reading the letter many years later that Brock had sent to my grandfather telling him that he would see me when I was about four years old and that I must not catch a chill and therefore must wear a vest, etc. Unfortunately that letter has now been lost. I cannot remember much before the first operation (the Brock Procedure) which took place in April 1954. Until after the operation I was not able to walk even a short distance without having to sit or squat.

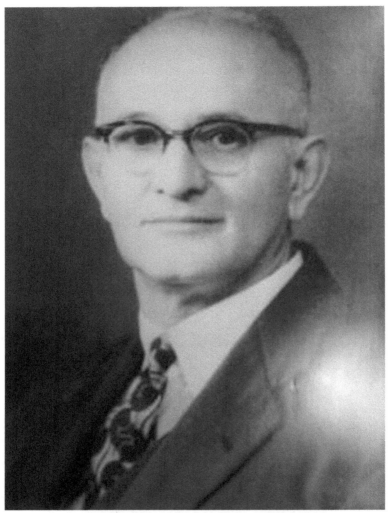
Dr Elchi Sorabjee, Xerxes grandfather who qualified at Guys in 1924, three years ahead of Brock.

Tom Treasure

The family came to London to see Sir Russell Brock at 2 Harley Street. Xerxes has a teddy bear with him and the family recalled that Brock had first put his stethoscope to the bear's chest and listened and told Xerxes that the bear seemed alright and that rather serious looking surgeon asked the little boy if he could now listen to his heart and he happily assented. Fallot's Tetralogy was diagnosed and Brock advised an operation. Xerxes' parents were told that there was a 50/50 chance that their little boy would not survive. Sir Russell Brock carried out the Brock Procedure in April 1954.

Xerxes continues – Just after the first operation I remember being in a clear plastic tent with various nurses coming in and out but I cannot remember my parents being there. However, I do recall my mother noticing a dramatic colour change in her son and commenting on this. My first memory after leaving hospital was going for a walk with my father along the bank of the Thames and seeing Tower Bridge rising to let a ship through. I was amazed by the ships funnel tilting back!

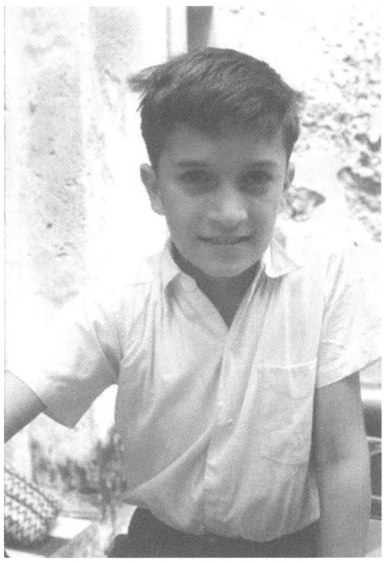

Xerxes at about 7 years old after his palliative operation in Guys Hospital by Brock.

DR. JOHN C. WINTELER

TELEPHONE
CONSULTING ROOMS, 23821 & 23822.
RESIDENCE, RIVERSIDE DRIVE 53165

COPY.

CORNER HOUSE
P.O. BOX 317
NAIROBI.

4th January, 1958.

Dear Dr. Campbell,

Xerxes Talati was brought to see me again on the 28th December. He is now 7 years of age and does anything and everything. His grandfather is a doctor and he tells me that sometimes Xerxes gets slight cyanosis on extreme exertion. I made him exert himself here and there was no cyanosis visible. He also gets a little dyspnoeic on exertion, but only on extreme exertion. He plays cricket with a soft ball and he swims in the sea. He has no cough, no fever and no swelling of the ankles at any time. There is finger-clubbing and no cyanosis. The apex beat was three inches from the mid-line; there was a systolic murmur and a thrill, loudest and most marked in the third and fourth left spaces; P2 was audible and there was a systolic murmur too, heard all over the precordium. His spleen was one fingerbreadth below the costal margin, but he lives at Zanzibar and he is taking anti-malarials. His cardiogram shows right ventricular preponderance; I enclose the copy; and an X-ray of his chest shows:-

"The apex is a little high and just overlaps the spine in the left oblique and the right ventricle shows slightly increased prominence in that view. The pulmonary arc remains slightly convex. The hilar vessels and pulmonary vascular markings do not appear abnormal."

The cardiothoracic picture is 9½ centimetres to 98. I must say he has done extremely well. I saw him first when he was nine months old in 1951 and all his relatives are delighted with the result.

With kind regards to you.

Yours sincerely,

JOHN C. WINTELER, M.D., M.R.C.P.

Dr. Maurice Campbell
Guy's Hospital, London.   Copy to Dr. F.S. Talati.

Letter from Xerxes doctor in Nairobi to Dr Campbell.

Three children growing up with part treated congenital heart disease

From 1954 the three children, Geraldine, John and Xerxes, then aged ten, six and four, were no longer deeply cyanosed and they were able to be much more active. As far as the Peacock Club is concerned that is the end of the historical account. For the children made better and in many cases only alive because of their palliative surgery, this was only the beginning of the rest of their lives with congenital heart disease. They have each written about their lives from 1954 to the present.

The lives of children with part treated congenital heart disease was commonly very eventful and for these three children it was known that if they were to have long lives, more surgery would be needed. Between them these three patients provide examples.

John Hunt from his palliative operation in 1954 to repair in 1961 and its aftermath

JH – I had to wait until I was 14 and admitted to Brompton on 9th October 1961 when Sir Russell (under my physician, Dr Paul Wood) carried out a secondary repair of Fallots Tetralogy. Prior to the operation my symptoms included fainting when standing for any length of time, eg. in church services, and this improved post operation. However there was a serious setback 24 hours after the surgery when I went in to rapid tachycardia and needed a tracheostomy and a mechanical respirator. About 14 days later the right lobe of the lung collapsed and I was opened up again to rewire the sternum. I was eventually discharged four months and nine days after being admitted.

My sister brought back something I had forgotten which was that after my 1961 operation I had a picture in the local newspaper of me with a garden spade under the heading of something like Miracle Boy! Overall, living with Congenital Heart Disease and siblings, I found on the one hand kept us apart in the sense of not being able to play games etc., but on the other hand bringing us closer together in perhaps a more meaningful sense.

Tom Treasure

The childhood part of the story might have ended there with the correction operation in December 1961 but exactly one year later 1962 when I was beginning to get over the operation and gain some confidence, I was playing with a friend at school when he punched me on my chest. I went in to rapid ventricular tachycardia at about 300 beats a minute with a lot of loss of blood from a haemorrhage (the cause of which still puzzles me and does not appear in my old reports). The local hospital in Northampton could not regulate the heart and after a few days I was rushed to London in an ambulance. It remains a mystery as to why I was not taken to my hospital at Brompton and it turned out to be nearly two weeks before dramatic corrective action was taken.

After initially being sent to the National Heart Hospital, I had ended up in Guys Hospital in a childrens ward and it being near Christmas I remember, from my semi-conscious state, that the children had decorated the ward with large letters saying Sir Brussell Rock! By some miracle (as you might guess – I needed quite a few, even at this stage in my life, to keep me going) Sir Russell just happened to walk by my bed as he was a consultant at Guys as well as being my surgeon at Brompton. Apparently he was furious that he had not been told of my dwindling state and immediately ordered a cardioversion. I remember quite vividly two large pads being placed on my chest and nothing else apart from suddenly feeling well and hungry! As the report of 27th December 1962 from Guys says, dramatically the heart rhythm changed from ventricular tachycardia to sinus rhythm. When I was referred to Dr Jane Somerville in1993 her report said that It was such a novel treatment at the time that it was written up in the Literature. I have since learned that the novel treatment was written up in *The Lancet* because at the time cardioversion had only been used at the time of actual operations and my case was the first to use it at a time other than during an operation.[99]

œsophageal lead (fig. 1), were present. Treatment with sedation, mersalyl, and digoxin was started, and the degree of heart-failure lessened. Quinidine sulphate by mouth and quinidine hydrochloride intravenously were administered during four days, and produced temporary slowing of the ventricular rate to 100 per minute with toxic symptoms. The arrhythmia persisted. It was therefore decided to use electrical countershock, after consultation with Sir Russell Brock, and this was applied by Mr. Donald Ross on Dec. 24. 400 volts were given externally over the long axis of the heart using alternating current from a ' Cardiac Recorders ' defibrillator; the patient was under general anæsthesia with nitrous oxide, oxygen, and thiopentone. Sinus rhythm (fig. 2) occurred, after a brief phase of nodal rhythm, in less than a minute. Thereafter the patient recovered uneventfully, and he has remained well and in sinus rhythm, taking quinidine sulphate 0·3 g. t.d.s.

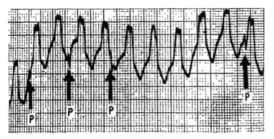

Fig. 1—Œsophageal lead showing ventricular tachycardia at 162 per minute. Atrial rate 91 per minute.

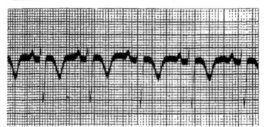

Fig. 2—Lead V₂ showing sinus rhythm restored following electrical countershock.

An extract from the publication in The Lancet about John Hunt who was the first patient to have an external electrical countershock to correct ventricular tachycardia.[99]

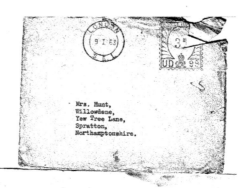

A letter to Johns mother from Russell Brock who was displeased that John had been sent to the National Heart Hospital rather than back to his care.

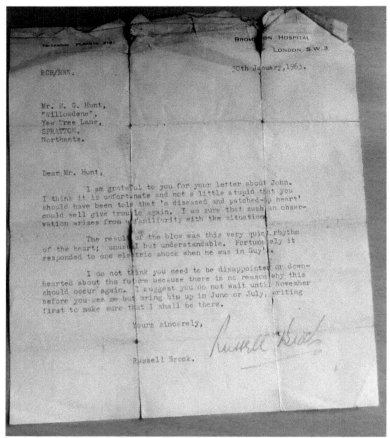

Following John Hunts terrifying experience of going from one hospital to another with his heart beating up to 200 times a minute, his distressed father wrote to Brock. Brock replied in this letter.

The second period over Christmas was a little more vague as I was still recovering from the second major surgery and its complications. The last period was ironically the one I remember the best – even though I was semi-conscious with ventricular tachycardia having had the playful blow to the chest at school on 14th December 1962 I referred to earlier. Apart from the dash in the ambulance from Northampton to London, my strongest memory of that time was lying in bed in Guys Hospital in the childrens ward with the decorations all around and the amazing luck of Sir Russell Brock discovering me there and giving me the gift of one of the first cardioversions in the world on Christmas day. I think Christmas is all about the miracle of Christs birth but that day I was giving thanks for my own re-birth!

From 1962 to the present day, life has been filled with work as a solicitor, travels to exotic countries on various conservation projects and generally learning what the world is all about. Medically the early operations were a great success and provided I used common sense in life style activities such as eating sensibly (vegetarian), no smoking and little alcohol with regular exercise, then I had very few negative effects from the congenital heart disease. However there is inevitably wear and tear in older hearts and the scarring tissue in the heart from early surgery has caused arrhythmias which needed attention. Therefore an ICD (pacemaker and defibrillator) was inserted in January 2005 following ventricular tachycardia and a new pulmonary valve implanted in July 2005. Ongoing treatment continues with the same expertise and care that I have become used to.

I would just like to express my eternal gratitude to the whole Brompton team who have done such marvellous work on me over the last 60 years and can only say that the NHS, which came into being the year I was born, has ensured that I have had, what I consider to be, the most caring, pioneering and expert surgeons and teams in the world!

The Heart Club

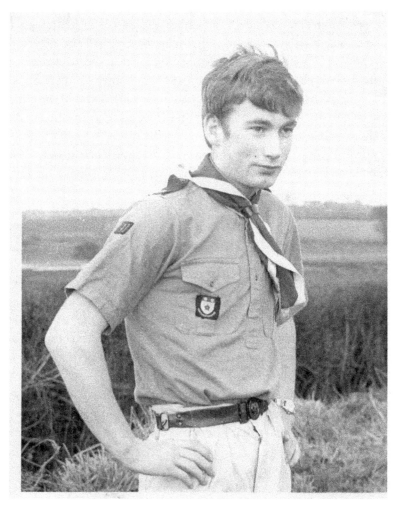

John Hunt in early 1966, three years after the ventricular tachycardia and electrical countershock.

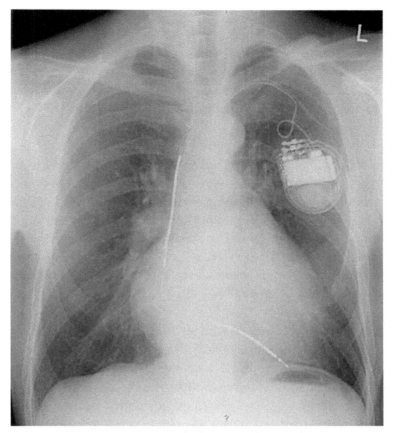

A recent X-ray of John Hunts chest with
his defibrillator and pacing leads.

The Heart Club

Xerxes Talati from palliative operation in 1954 to repair in 1967

XT – After returning to Zanzibar in 1954, I started school in a kindergarten. There was no paper available and so everything was learnt by writing on a slate with chalk. After that my junior school days were in Zanzibar. I still could not run for more than twenty yards before getting very breathless and squatting, but that did not worry me as I caught up with the others as soon as I recovered.

My senior schooling was at a boarding school in Ely in Cambridgeshire. There was a definite change in the average temperature especially as there was a lack of hot water and heating in the school but all the boys became used to it quite quickly. I was exempt from sport but had to hide my disappointment as I became breathless on exertion. This was demonstrated quite easily at the beginning of every term when I had to carry my case up a short hill from the railway station to the school. This caused a change of complexion from pink to blue accompanied by nausea.

Whilst at school in Ely I used to go to see Sir Russell (later Lord) Brock for a yearly review in the Christmas holidays. In December 1966 Brock noticed a change and became concerned. He had always told me that he would have to perform a second operation before I was 20 years of age. At boarding school in Ely, Cambridgeshire, I joined in with the other boys in games and was not noticeably handicapped, but as time went by I fell behind on cross country runs and friends would hang back for me.

In the school holidays Xerxes would go to see Sir Russell. He was alone on his visit to 2 Harley Street in 1967. Brock didn't like what he found on examining Xerxes heart and told him to go immediately to Guy's Hospital for an x-ray and to bring it straight back. The distance was about four miles and Brock said 'Don't go on the tube, take a taxi'. Seventeen year-old Xerxes had only his pocket money which would not stretch to a taxi. Brock took out his wallet and gave him enough money for the taxi. Xerxes came back with the x-ray which confirmed Brock's fears.

Tom Treasure

FROM
LORD BROCK.

2, HARLEY STREET,
CAVENDISH SQUARE, W.1.

5th December, 1975.

Mrs.Talati of 592, Southcroft Road, London, S.W.16.

I have known this lady since 1954 when I did an operation on her son, Xerxes Talati, for a serious heart condition. This operation had to be revised in 1957 and he is now completely cured.

His father died soon after the second operation and his widowed mother returned to Kenya but her son continued at school in England and subsequently has been studying at University College, London. He obtained a degree in chemistry and is now in the middle of taking a course of a University degree in dental surgery which he expects to complete in 1978.

His mother is on a visit from Kenya but her wish is to stay in England with her son. I understand she has adequate means of support and has no family connections in Kenya.

I believe that she will satisfy the requirements to be allowed to stay in England and I strongly recommend that she should be allowed to do so. She is a very nice lady and I am sure will be a credit to this country.

Brock

Lord Brock, M.S., F.R.C.S..

Xerxes father died suddenly in London soon after Xerxes second operation. Lord Brock wrote to support his mothers wish to stay in England with her only son.

The Heart Club

Both Xerxes and his mother recall their parting on the night before the operation. Xerxes stood at the window of his room in Nuffield House, the private wing of Guy's Hospital. His mother remembers looking back from Guy's 'park' to see Xerxes at the window waving to her. Xerxes was terrified but stood waving to give his mother the comfort of knowing that he was alright.

Brock operated to close the ventricular septal defect and complete the correction of Fallot's Tetralogy in July 1967. Xerxes chest was reopened in the night to deal with excessive bleeding. The problem was solved and he recovered well.

Xerxes writes – This total repair was performed in July 1967 at the age of 17, and I had a very successful outcome. I was then able to take part in sporting events such as cross country running but was more successful in the 100-yard sprint.

Xerxes father died suddenly of a ruptured aneurysm before the family left London. One of the acts of personal kindness towards them which Brock's patients remember was that Lord Brock (as he had become) wrote in support of his mother being able to stay in Britain.

Geraldine West from palliation at the second attempt in 1954, through two episodes of endocarditis, to a repair operation in 1979

I was aware from quite a young age that my condition had an adverse effect on my siblings. I was a needy child through all of my elder brother and sisters formative years and have no doubt that this contributed to her anxieties and insecurities and his behaviour – he was a very naughty boy! My younger sister too has told me that she experienced a lack of parental supervision and got away with things she should not have been allowed to get away with like frequent truanting from school. My younger brother, a quiet gentle artist, was possibly the least affected since, by the time he was four, I was well.

Life at secondary school was uneventful. I was very pleased at not being allowed to do PE or games, but a little disappointed at not being allowed to go on school outings or journeys. School seemed to me to be a place where you went to have fun rather than to do any work. Listening to adults talking above my head and my own understanding of my health, I knew my life was to be a short one, so there was not much point in striving for a good education or a career. This was a regret in later life that I endeavoured to correct, taking O Levels in Maths and English and gaining various adult teaching and training qualifications.

Three weeks after my 16th birthday I got a job as a shorthand typist in a city firm of tea merchants and when I was 17 I met my future husband. We married in the spring of 1965. Early the following year I became ill. Cold and shivering and hot and perspiring in turns, a constant throbbing headache, aching limbs and distressing night sweats – I thought I had a bad dose of flu and determined to fight it – and fight it I did, taking Beechams Powders at frequent intervals and dragging myself around. I had not heard of endocarditis and neither, it seemed, had my GP. After almost two months, my mother, increasingly anxious about me, arranged for me to see my childhood doctor. It was Good Friday. Within ten minutes she had arranged for me to be admitted to The Middlesex and had called for an ambulance.

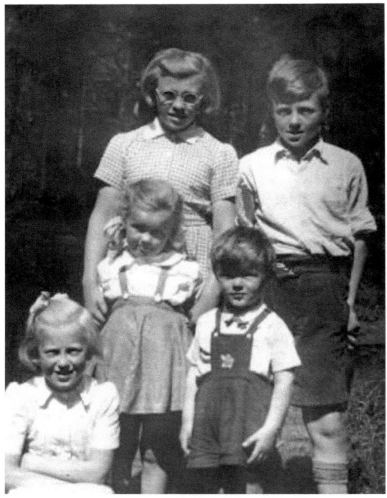
Geraldine at the front, the middle child of five.

Tom Treasure

After eight weeks of four-hourly penicillin and streptomycin injections, not only was I no better, but now had pleurisy. Dr (Walter) Somerville said that they would keep on keeping on, but I was exhausted and distressed and knew I was losing this battle for my life. Shortly after his ward round, a volunteer hospital visitor stopped by my bed. I dont remember exactly what she said to me but it was along the lines of its up to you, stop feeling sorry for yourself, pull yourself together, do battle with this illness. She inspired me to do just that. Within a few days my temperature – at last – stabilised and two weeks later I went home.

It was some months before I was well enough to return to work and since we were managing without my income, we decided to explore the possibility of having a child. Dr Walter Somerville, who had been my consultant at The Middlesex for some years, gave me the go-ahead and in 1967 I had a daughter, followed by a second daughter in 1970. Apart from extreme tiredness (and migraine, which continues to be a nuisance) both pregnancies and births were trouble-free. As time went on, with two young children and a job, life became more of a struggle for me. I knew that I could have further surgery but I was putting it off, wanting my children to be older. But then I had endocarditis again. I was taken ill at work, knew straight away what it was, went home, phoned my GP and was admitted to the Brook Hospital in Woolwich the next morning. It was the 5th November 1978.

This time I knew the score and once Id got over my dismay at having this illness again, I focussed all my strength on fighting it. For the next six weeks I mostly slept and ate! I went home on Christmas Eve, returning to hospital each morning for doses of penicillin and streptomycin. On New Years Day, a young doctor I had not seen before came to administer these antibiotics. He told me he had been at a party all night. Leaving the hospital that morning I felt ill and for the next three months struggled with vertigo. I was told by the pathologist that streptomycin was the cause and that it was likely that I had been given an overdose.

When I next saw Dr Somerville, he spoke of further surgery and when I again hesitated, he took my hand in both of his and said simply I think its time. Three weeks later, I was back in The Middlesex – Holmes Sellors ward

The Heart Club

this time, appropriately. Mr Sturridge operated and returned me to health. *He tied the Blalock shunt, patched the ventricular septal defect and completed the repair of Fallot's Tetralogy.*

Apart from arrhythmia for which I had ablations in 1996 and is troublesome at times, I have been in good health and lead a normal life. I worked until I was 67, go to the gym, swim, walk and if need be can even run upstairs. I am not on any medication. Overall my life has been enriched by this condition. It has made me appreciate each day and be tolerant of others.

As a doctor I was trained to relate clinical histories dispassionately in so far as I can. For these three individuals, telling their medical stories and remembering their operations cannot be separated from their sentiments and the totality of their lives. These are their lives and we conclude the chapter with some of their own reflections.

Xerxes Talati – After finishing school, I did a degree course in Chemistry and financed myself by earning money as a hospital porter at The Middlesex and Westminster Hospitals. I then managed to gain admission at the UCH Dental School and qualified in 1979. Whilst at university I had a fairly normal life and played hockey for UCH. After qualifying I worked in the Maxillo-Facial departments at Guys and Poole General Hospitals in order to gain some surgical experience. I was offered a registrars post at Guys but decided to go into General Dental Practice instead where I stayed for nearly 30 years before retiring. I did go into atrial flutter and had a cardiac ablation in June last year (2016). I am now back into sinus rhythm. So far so good!

Geraldine West – From the start, I have been blessed with good fortune. From my much loved and loving parents who were so courageous on my behalf; the skilled surgeons Sir Thomas Holmes Sellors and Marvin Sturridge; my consultants Walter Somerville, Howard Swanton and now Fiona Walker, Dr McGonagall at the Brook, Dr Eileen Gorman my childhood GP and GP Dr Sutton; the nursing and other staff at The Middlesex and the Brook; Dr Campbells cousin, the hospital visitor and my family and friends. And lastly, my heart – a true warrior! They have all played their part in my survival and I thank them.

Tom Treasure

John Hunt – Heart problems touch most people or their relatives and friends at some time in their lives and stories of we patients will hopefully add a bit of realism to the hard facts of the Peacock Club: the development of the early history of heart surgery including methods of measuring the circulation and oxygen concentrations, cooling to protect the heart and the brain during surgery, the heart lung machine. We three patients present not only a theoretical admiration of scientific and medical progress but a heart-felt gratitude to those pioneers whom we were lucky enough to encounter at the crucial times in our lives.

Biographical Notes: List 1

The Peacock Club members and guests.

Abrahams, Derek Gordon (1918–1981) was cardiology senior registrar at the National Heart Hospital (1949–52) when he attended the Club as a guest in December 1949 with a group of cardiologists including Paul Wood and Walter Somerville. Previously Derek Abrahams worked at the Special Unit for Juvenile Rheumatism, Canadian Red Cross Memorial Hospital, Taplow from where he wrote on the ECG in rheumatic fever.[110] Apparently Wood did not think highly of Derek Abrahams. In 1952 he went to the USA on a travelling fellowship returning to the London Hospital. He then went to Ibadan, Nigeria, in 1956 and then Australia in 1963 to the University of New South Wales and later to Royal North Shore Hospital, Sydney.
Q: Cambridge and St Georges 1945; MRCP 1947; MD 1950; FRCP 1979.
http://munksroll.rcplondon.ac.uk/Biography/Details/7

Allanby, Kenneth Derwent (1922–2002) was at the first meeting of the Club and attended in the first year while in a junior positon in the department of medicine. He wrote on circulation times in congenital heart disease[111] and with other Club members on pulmonary stenosis[112] and pulmonary atresia[113]. Kenneth Allanby was appointed house physician at Guys in November 1945. Later he worked for Paul Wood at the Brompton and was senior registrar to Evan Bedford at The Middlesex. He came back as a visitor in March 1951. He returned to Guys as senior assistant in the department of medicine. For 30 years from 1961 he was a consultant physician in Peterborough.
Q: The Middlesex Hospital 1945; MRCP 1947, MD (University Medal) 1951.
http://munksroll.rcplondon.ac.uk/Biography/Details/5318

Ashmore, Philip Godfrey (1926–2011) was a paediatric surgeon, recorded as attending the Club in January 1956. Philip Ashmore graduated in Toronto

The Heart Club

and influenced by the Canadian cardiovascular surgeon Bill Mustard, in 1954 he gained an overseas fellowship to work with Russell Brock, visiting Great Ormond Street weekly to be with David Waterston. He returned to Vancouver and developed paediatric and adult cardiac surgery there.
Q: Toronto 1948
http://www.bcmj.org/obituaries/dr-phillip-godfrey-ashmore

Baker, Charles Gaffney (1907–1969) was a regular at the Club meetings. He wrote and contributed on many papers related to the work of the Club.[63;75;103;114-121] Charles Baker was registrar at Guys and editor of *Guy's Hospital Gazette* 1933–34 and was appointed to Selly Oaks Hospital in Birmingham. He served in the army during WW2 and was welcomed back to Guys as assistant physician to Guys Hospital and sub-dean of the medical school in 1946. He was appointed assistant physician to the Cardiac Department from September 1949. He was Warden of the College from 1947, an appointment peculiar to Guys and he often entertained the Club in the Wardens House. Willie Mann, a Guys physician, wrote in Munks Roll of Bakers sociability, wide learning, and his many friends. He was undoubtedly important in cementing the Club membership together.
Q: Guys Hospital LDS RCS 1930; MB BS 1935; MRCP 1936; MD 1937; FRCP 1948
http://munksroll.rcplondon.ac.uk/Biography/Details/191

Barrett, Norman Rupert (1903–1979) attended the Club in March and September 1950.
Barrett was a thoracic surgeon at St Thomas Hospital. He had written a paper with Raymond Daley about a surgical means of increasing blood flow to the lungs in cyanotic heart disease using pleural adhesions.[122] At the meeting in September 1950, also attended by Bill Cleland, Denton Cooley and James ONeill, Pasty Barrett asked about the nature of the Peacock club, possibly seeking membership, and in reply Maurice Campbell indicated from the chair that it was essentially a Guys club. Mr Barrett did not take well to cardiac surgery but was a prominent thoracic surgeon well-known for the description of Barretts oesophagus. I was surgical registrar when he was admitted to St Thomas Hospital for a prostatectomy in 1975.
Q: St Thomass 1928; FRCS 1930; MCh 1931
http://livesonline.rcseng.ac.uk/biogs/E006299b.htm

Tom Treasure

Bates, Michael (1917–1985) attended the Club in February 1950 when Russell Brock was reporting on his exchange visit in 1949 to Johns Hopkins. Mr Bates was in training with Oswald Tubbs and Russell Brock at the Brompton at the time. He made some sorties into cardiac surgery with his colleagues Raymond Hurt but they did not persevere with open heart surgery. He was thoracic surgeon to the North Middlesex Hospital where they continued with mitral valvotomy for some years.

Q: St Bartholomews Hospital 1941; FRCS 1949

http://livesonline.rcseng.ac.uk/biogs/E007111b.htm

Baylis, John Horton (1921–present) was a medical registrar at Guys when he attended the Club in February 1955 to present work on coarctation as part of Campbells series of studies on the natural history and prognosis of congenital heart disease.[104]

John Baylis wrote papers with Maurice Campbell.[104;123;124] He was later registrar at the Brompton and senior registrar at Kings. He was a consultant physician in Bedford until his retirement.

Q: Guys 1947; MRCP 1951; FRCP 1971

Brain, Robert Henry Field (1914–1993) attended the Club once as a member in November 1952. Robert Brain came to Guys from Birmingham as a thoracic surgeon. He was doing some cardiac operations as I knew from being his house surgeon in 1970-71 but his work was predominately non-cardiac thoracic surgery. There was one cardiac case listed for him during the three months I was his house surgeon, an atrial septal defect, but in the event the operation was started and completed by the Terry McEnany the exchange senior registrar from the MGH, Boston, USA.

Q: Birmingham 1937; FRCS 1940

http://livesonline.rcseng.ac.uk/biogs/E007838b.htm

Brinton, Wilfred Danvers (1911–1984) was a senior medical registrar at Guys and a regular attender of the Club from the first meeting until February 1951. He wrote with other members on pulmonary stenosis[113] and Ebsteins disease[117] and as sole author on primary pulmonary hypertension.[125] His important personal contribution was a series of papers about haematological changes in cyanotic heart disease and changes with surgical relief.[126-128]

219

The Heart Club

Dr Brinton was in the RAMC 1939 to 1945. In 1950 he was appointed consultant physician to the Winchester Group of Hospitals.

Q: Oxford 1938; MRCP 1946; DM 1950; FRCP 1967

http://munksroll.rcplondon.ac.uk/Biography/Details/553

Brock, Russell Claude (1903–1980) convened the first meeting for the Club and wrote prolifically during its lifetime.[1;30;59;63;98;103;105;114;115;118;129-157] Russell Brock received a Rockefeller Foundation Travelling Fellowship from The Medical Research Council 1930–31 announced in the *Times*, June 20, 1930. He was editor of *Guy's Hospital Reports* which included documentation of the work of the Club members, often in detail and at length. Brock was knighted in 1954 and became Lord Brock of Wimbledon in 1965. A sentence in the Minutes which is picked up as capturing Brock by readers who knew him appeared in March 1951: Mr Brock remarked that it was easy to go on finding objections, the thing was to get on with the job. I met him in the operating theatres as student in 1967 and again when I assisted him with a lobectomy in 1970 when I was house surgeon to the Thoracic Unit at Guys.

Q: Guys 1927; FRCS 1929; MS 1931; FRCP 1965

http://livesonline.rcseng.ac.uk/biogs/E000235b.htm

Brotmacher, Leon (1925–not found) was a Research Fellow at Guys when he attended as a member of the Club in January and March 1956, the last meetings of the club. He may well have attended earlier. He published with Dennis Deuchar[158] Peter Fleming[159;160] and with Maurice Campbell on the natural history of ventricular septal defect.[106] In 1957 he published work on squatting, a consistent feature of Fallots Tetralogy, from Guys as part of his PhD thesis.[161;162] Before going to Guys, Brotmacher had done military service in Somalia and published a study of its traditional medical practice.[163] He came to Guys from Cardiff Infirmary and went on in 1957 to be senior medical registrar in the Royal United Hospital in Bath. He emigrated to USA/Canada according to the records of the Royal Grammar School, High Wycombe.

Q: St Marys 1946; MRCP 1950

http://www.rgs.saund.co.uk/rgsawards.html

Tom Treasure

Brown, Michael Meredith (1918–2009) attended the Club as a member from December 1949 to March 1950. He was a guest in May 1951 when he was a consultant thoracic surgeon at St Helier Hospital, Carshalton.
Q: Cambridge 1942; FRCS 1944
http://livesonline.rcseng.ac.uk/biogs/E001020b.htm

Brunnen, Peter Lance (1910–2000) attended as a member in October 1952 when he was a cardiovascular research fellow with Mr Brock 1951-1952. In 1953 he published his experiments on aortic grafting carried out with Brock.[79] Brunnen became a consultant thoracic surgeon in Aberdeen and worked further on aneurysms.[164]
Q: Aberdeen 1939; FRCS England and Edinburgh 1948
http://livesonline.rcseng.ac.uk/biogs/E009057b.htm

Bywaters, Eric George Lapthorne (1910–2003) attended the Club in March 1952 to join a discussion on rheumatic fever. Dr Bywaters had a prizewinning career including a Rockefeller Travelling Fellowship in 1937 spent at MGH, Boston. When he attended, he was the director of the research unit at the Canadian Red Cross Memorial Hospital Taplow from where he published research on rheumatic fever.[165-168] He was later consultant physician and Professor of Rheumatology at the Royal Postgraduate Medical School.
Q: The Middlesex 1933; MRCP 1937; FRCP 1950
http://munksroll.rcplondon.ac.uk/Biography/Details/5148

Campbell, John Maurice Hardman (1891–1973) was physician in charge of the cardiac department at Guys and a physician to the National Hospital for Diseases of the Heart. He chaired the second meeting in June 1948 and most of the subsequent ones. Campbell had the highest number of attendances at the Club meetings for which names were recorded in the Minutes. There is no record of any further meetings after his retirement. Shortly before the first meeting he had written up the Guys experience with the Blalock–Taussig operation for relief of cyanotic heart disease, the earlier ones by Alfred Blalock himself at Guys.[19] Presciently he wrote concerning the natural history of congenital heart disease Soon the physicians who are advising operation will have no experience of its natural course without this. It seems that someone who has lived through this period of change should try to collect what he can before it is too late. True to his word he wrote a series of papers doing exactly that.[106-108;169-174] During the years of the Club he authored many papers often with other Club members on all forms of congenital heart disease.[23;27;28;59;106;112;113;120;123;124;136;139;175-190] With Evan Bedford he was a first editor of the *BHJ* in 1938. He retired from active practice in 1956 but his contributions continued afterwards.

Q: Oxford and Guys 1916; MRCP and MD 1921; FRCP 1929.
http://munksroll.rcplondon.ac.uk/Biography/Details/737

Carnegie, David Michael (1917–2006) was an anaesthetist to Guys and the Evelina Hospital. He attended the meeting in March 1951 concerning selective angiography. In June 1951 Carnegie published a paper on 172 cases that underwent angiocardiography at Guys for congenital heart disease rejecting the view that it was a simple and harmless procedure.[72] His three fellow anaesthetists, Phillip Helliwell, Andrew Hutton and Ernest Rink were acknowledged and a full account of the problems they encountered was given. As house surgeon to Donald Ross I was in the operating theatre with him each week for three months in 1971.

Q: Guys 1943; DA 1947; FFA RCS 1953

Channell, Gerald Dalton (1911–1950) was assistant lecturer in anatomy and a regular attender at the Club until his last appearance in February 1950. He wrote on Ebsteins disease with Club members.[117] Gerald Channell won the Hilton Dissection Prize in 1933 and after a house surgeons job at Guys in 1938 he was appointed Demonstrator in Anatomy at Cambridge. After war service as Surgeon Lieutenant-Commander in the Royal Navy he returned to Guys and was appointed full-time demonstrator in anatomy in July 1946 and published studies in human anatomy.[191-193] He became interested in congenital deformities of the heart and was attracted to surgery. In a footnote to a subsequent publication Wilfred Brinton and Maurice Campbell wrote [Channells] knowledge of anatomy and embryology made him an ideal colleague for this work and the measurements of the earlier cases were mostly his. His death in an explosion at the Brompton Hospital ... was a tragic loss.[185]

Q: Cambridge and Guys 1936; FRCS 1949
http://livesonline.rcseng.ac.uk/biogs/E005587b.htm

Tom Treasure

Chesterman, Judson Tyndale (1903–1987) was consultant cardiothoracic surgeon at the City General Hospital in Sheffield and attended the Club as a guest in November 1950. Chesterman was prize-winner and gold medallist as a student in Bristol and had accolades from the College of Surgeons. He published on cardiac surgical topics during the time of the Club.[194-197]
Q: Bristol 1927; FRCS 1930; MRCP 1932
http://livesonline.rcseng.ac.uk/biogs/E007155b.htm

Cleland, William Paton (1912–2005) was on the surgical staff at the Brompton when he attended the Club as a guest in March and September 1950. Bill Cleland had come from Australia to Kings College Hospital in 1938 to be a resident medical officer. Service in KCHs wartime base in Horton, Surrey generated an interest in surgery. He took the FRCS examination and in 1948 went to the Brompton and worked with Russell Brock, Arthur Tudor Edwards and Clement Price Thomas. He was a consultant at the Brompton, Kings College Hospital and the Hammersmith Hospital. At Hammersmith Denis Melrose developed a heart-lung machine[198] which, with Hugh Bentall and the cardiologist Arthur Hollman, Cleland took to Moscow in 1959 operating there on five children with congenital heart disease.
Q: Adelaide 1934; MRCP 1939; FRCS 1946; FRCP 1967
http://livesonline.rcseng.ac.uk/biogs/E000162b.htm

Cooley, Denton Arthur (1920–2016) attended the Club as a guest in September 1950.
Cooley graduated from Johns Hopkins, Baltimore where he worked with Alfred Blalock. In 1950 he went to the Brompton to work with Russell Brock. He published prolifically when he returned to America and was an early adopter of surgery for mitral stenosis.[199] He was a highly skilled, fast, high volume surgeon, naming his private practice the Texas Heart Institute.
Q: Johns Hopkins
https://en.wikipedia.org/wiki/Denton_Cooley

Cosh, John Arthur (1915–2005) was a medical registrar in Bristol when he attended the Club as a guest in January 1951. Dr Cosh graduated from St Thomas Hospital. He went to Bristol in 1948 where he trained and published on cardiology.[200] In 1957 he was appointed as consultant physician to the Bath area and then moved via rheumatology into herbal medicine and then the Bristol Cancer Help Centre.

Q:Cambridge and St Thomass MRCS LRCP and MB BChir 1940; MRCP 1947; MD 1951; FRCP 1964

http://munksroll.rcplondon.ac.uk/Biography/Details/5705

Daley, Raymond (1917–1989) was chief assistant at the National Heart Hospital when he attended in September 1950 and October 1951. At this second meeting he contributed to discussions about pulmonary venous and capillary pressure measurements. After the war, Raymond Daley had been senior registrar to John McMichael (later Sir John) at the Royal Postgraduate Medical School. He was awarded a Rockefeller fellowship to study at Harvard and Johns Hopkins. There he met Richard Gorlin who later worked with him at St Thomas Hospital after Daley was appointed to the cardiac department in 1951. They published extensively in this era.[122;201;202]

Q: Cambridge and St Thomass 1941, MRCP 1942, MD 1946, FRCP 1956

http://munksroll.rcplondon.ac.uk/Biography/Details/1126

Darke, Christopher Sydney (1913–1991) was a medical registrar at the Brompton when he attended with a group of cardiologists in December 1949. Dr Darke was appointed consultant in Sheffield in 1950.

Q Guys 1936 MRCP 1938; MD 1939; FRCP 1962

http://munksroll.rcplondon.ac.uk/Biography/Details/1143

De Navasquez, Sigiberto Jose (1905/6-1971) was Reader in Pathology at Guys on the one occasion he was known to have attended the Club in January 1952. He told the Club that there was much material for study in the biopsies of the lung and auricular appendix which had been routinely collected during operations for mitral stenosis. John Enticknap, Benjamin Milstein and Charles Baker subsequently published from this collection of pathological material.[73;74;75] Siggi De Navasquez was born in Saõ Paulo, Brazil. He worked in bacteriology, morbid anatomy and experimental pathology. He was made Professor in 1965.

Q: Guys 1928; DTM&H 1929; MD 1934

Obituary *BMJ* 13th March 1971 P.612

Tom Treasure

Deuchar, Dennis Charles (1924–1977) was on the medical staff at Guys and as one of the younger members of the Club attended regularly from December 1949 to March 1953. A year after qualification he began work developing the cardiac catheterisation laboratory with Eddie Holling and George Zak, building some of the equipment himself. He was a founder member of the Biological Engineering Society. He spent a year as a fellow at Johns Hopkins. He published regularly with other members to the Club.[27;28;78;158;203-208] He was appointed assistant physician to the cardiac department at Guys in 1958. Dr Deuchar taught me when I was a clinical medical student 1967-1970. He succeeded Charles Baker and Ralph Kauntze as physician-in-charge in 1971.
Q: Guys 1948, MRCP 1951, MD 1952.
http://munksroll.rcplondon.ac.uk/Biography/Details/1245

Dow, John Dickson (1916–2007) was appointed consultant radiologist at Guys in 1953 and invited to become a member of the Club in February 1955. Dr Dows previous work had been on venography.[209-211] I was taken by Donald Ross to be shown coronary angiograms by Dow in 1971 while I was a house surgeon.
Q: Glasgow 1940; DMRD Eng 1946; FFR 1953; MRCP Ed 1967; FRCP Ed 1970
https://www.rcpe.ac.uk/obituary/dr-john-dickson-dow-frcp-edin

Douglas, William Keith (1917–2015) was probably a junior in the surgical team when he attended in March 1952 and was listed as a member of the Club. Mr Douglas was later a cardiothoracic surgeon at Wythenshawe Hospital Manchester.
Q: Cambridge 1943, FRCS 1950, MChir 1958
http://livesonline.rcseng.ac.uk/biogs/E008076b.htm

Dubost, Charles (1914–1991) from LHôpital Broussais, Paris attended the Club in February 1951. By this time Dubost was publishing prolifically and was already a prominent figure in cardiac surgery. He is credited with the first resection and interposition homograft for an abdominal aortic aneurysm performed a little after his visit on 29th March 1951.[212] Russell Brock did his first operation on a thoracic aortic aneurysm in November 1951 and at the same time resected a coarctation.[141]
https://fr.wikipedia.org/wiki/Charles_Dubost_(chirurgien)

The Heart Club

Earl, Christopher Joseph (1925–2012) was at the meetings in June and July 1948. He would have been a house physician at the time and hence was entered in the Minutes as Mr Earl. Earl was later consultant neurologist at the National Hospital, Queen Square and various London teaching hospitals.
Q: Guys 1948; MRCP 1950; MD 1951; FRCP 1964
http://munksroll.rcplondon.ac.uk/Biography/Details/6497

Enticknap, John Brandon (1922–2012) was a junior on the Guys medical staff when attending the Club at least four times between March 1952 and March 1954. At the meeting in the Wardens House (Charles Bakers residence) in March 1952 he presented post mortem findings later published.[73] Later in the year (November) again in Bakers house the meeting was devoted to a presentation of the pulmonary changes in mitral stenosis, material also later published.[74;75] He published other reports of cardiac pathology.[213;214] Enticknap was appointed to East Ham Memorial Hospital in 1954 and Whipps Cross in 1971 as a consultant pathologist. He was involved in forensic pathology, service organisation and research in ischaemic heart disease.
Q: Charing Cross 1945; MD 1952; FRCPath 1966
Obituary: BMJ 2013;346:168

Fleming, Peter Robert (1924–2002) was registrar in the cardiac department (1955–57) when he attended the Club as a member in December 1955 and March 1956. He was regularly in the operating theatre when Russell Brock was operating and he reported five patients of Brocks in 1956.[153;156] The precedence for descriptions of subaortic left ventricular obstruction has been contested but Brock appears to have a reasonable claim to have observed and recorded this condition first. With his surgeon contemporary Leon Brotmacher, Peter Fleming did clinical experiments in intravascular pressure measurement.[159;215] Peter Fleming went on to the Westminster Hospital, continued his interest in clinical measurement and worked closely with the surgeon Charles Drew.
Q: The Middlesex Hospital 1948; MRCP 1949; MD 1952; FRCP 1968
http://munksroll.rcplondon.ac.uk/Biography/Details/5256

Foxon, George Eric Howard (1908–1979) was Professor in the Department of Biology at Guys 1948-72 and made one recorded appearance in January 1949 for a talk on cardiac embryology by Rupert Willis. He talked to the Club about work he had published in *Nature*[216] and the *Journal of Anatomy*[217], contradicting the belief that the spiral septum of the frog separately streamed desaturated and oxygenated blood. He made the point that theorising about function from anatomical observations was unreliable. Foxon had also published technical papers about cineradiography[218;219] from the department of zoology University College Cardiff where he worked between 1937 and 1948. Both the observation and the method were of interest to the Peacock Club members.

Queens College Cambridge; BA 1930; 1st Class Hons Natural Science Tripos Pt II 1931

http://www.kingscollections.org/catalogues/kclca/collection/f/10fo90-1

Fry, Ian Kelsey (1923–present) was at the first meeting. He was Russell Brocks houseman.

While a houseman he wrote on thoracic topics, particularly complications of dental extraction.[220;221] His father, Sir William Kelsey Fry, was a leading dental surgeon and a governor of Guys.

Q: Guys 1948, DMRD 1961, DM Oxf 1962, FFR 1963

Gardner, Frances Violet (1913–1989) was on the medical staff at the Royal Free Hospital, when she attended in May 1949 and demonstrated full sized angiocardiograms made at the hospital. She is considered to have introduced the technique in Britain on return from a travelling fellowship in the USA.[222] She published papers with members of the club.[113;223] Frances Gardner was a consultant at the Royal Free for 32 years and dean from 1962–75.

Q: Royal Free 1940; MRCP 1943; MD 1943; FRCP 1952; FRCS 1983

http://munksroll.rcplondon.ac.uk/Biography/Details/1701

The Heart Club

Gorlin, Richard (1926?-1997) made one recorded attendance as a guest on 25 November 1952. He was a fellow at St Thomas Hospital with Raymond Daley and published with him.[202] He is known for the Gorlin formula to calculate the size of the orifice of the mitral valve, which he published in 1951.[224]

Q: Harvard

http://circ.ahajournals.org/content/97/8/715

http://www.nytimes.com/1997/10/18/nyregion/richard-gorlin-71-cardiologist-devised-diagnostic-method.html

Graham, John Wedgewood (1921-1985) came to Guys in 1949 for the fellowship course and attended the Club in March and April 1951 and again in November 1951 when he showed a specimen of a lung A.V. fistula in a meeting held in the library of the Pathology Department. He co-authored a case report with Russell Brock of a homograft replacement of a coarctation and aneurysm of the thoracic aorta, an operation done in November 1951.[141] John Graham worked as a surgical registrar in Birmingham, King Edward VII Hospital, Ealing and St Marks. He returned to Australia in 1954 and introduced vascular surgery at St Georges Hospital, Kogarah in 1960.

Q: Sydney 1944; FRCS 1950; FRACS 1956.

http://livesonline.rcseng.ac.uk/biogs/E007289b.htm

Hill, Ian Macdonald (1919–2007) was Russell Brocks senior registrar from 1947 and was one of the most regular members of the Club. He hand-wrote a number of the Minutes. He published less than the others making a single author paper in the *British Journal of Surgery* 1953 on A method of angiocardiography notable.[51] Ian Hill appears to have done the bulk of the clinical interventional work of angiocardiography as a junior surgeon. Ian Hill thanked Campbell and Brock for referring the cases, Dr Tom Hills for his help, Geoffrey Reynolds for the continuous ECGs and Ernest Rink, Philip Helliwell, Mike Hutton and David Carnegie for giving the anaesthetics. The syringes were made for me by Messrs. A. L. Hawkins of 15 New Cavendish Street, W1. He acknowledged and cited his colleagues papers[30;72;115;130;131;177;225-227] but was not an author on them. Long authors lists were not common then as they are now and it was this observation that led to the author network analysis that follows these Biographical Notes. Ian Hill was appointed consultant surgeon at Barts in 1950 at the age of 31. He continued to attend the Club until 1955.

Q: St Bartholomews 1942; FRCS 1944; MS 1945

http://livesonline.rcseng.ac.uk/biogs/E000558b.htm

Hills, Thomas Henry (1911–1974) was director of the diagnostic radiology unit and was a regular attender from September 1948 to March 1951 appearing a dozen times. He wrote numerous papers with other Club members.[71;177;225;226;228;229] Hills regularly presented angiocardiograms to the Club and in 1951 purchased a Fairchild roll film camera, previously used by the US Airforce for aerial reconnaissance during the war which was fitted beneath an ordinary fluorography table. This produced films of 9.5x9.5 inches at 2 per second, suitable for the young and adolescent heart and which caused anguish to the radiographers hand processing them in the old manual processors of that era.[230] This equipment made selective angiography possible.

http://www.bshr.org.uk/journals/018%20RHHCT%20Journal%2018%202002.pdf

Q: Cambridge and Guys 1937; DMRE 1940

https://www.ncbi.nlm.nih.gov/pmc/articles/PMC1444224/pdf/bmjcred00486-0096.pdf

Holling, Herbert Edward (1908–2000) was on the staff of Guys Clinical Research Unit when he began to regularly attend the Club from the first meeting until April 1951 and may well have attended often after then. Eddie Holling had a prize-winning undergraduate career in Sheffield and went to Bostons Peter Bent Brigham Hospital for two years and came from there to work at Guys with Ronald Grant on the peripheral circulation. He was central to the cardiovascular measuring and imaging which under pinned the work of the Club. In the paper reporting the first 100 mitral valvotomies the acknowledgment reads: The Guys group are particularly indebted to Dr H. E. Holling of the Medical Research Council Unit.[118] Holling published several papers related to the work of the club.[100;101;231-235] Eddie Holling developed a liking for America during his fellowship and returned permanently to Pennsylvania as a physician.

Q: Sheffield 1932; MRCP 1936; MD

http://munksroll.rcplondon.ac.uk/Biography/Details/6462

Hume. Mr Hume was recorded as attending the Club on two occasions, March and April 1949. My searches have revealed no convincing match.

The Heart Club

Hunter. Mr Hunter was recorded as attending the Club once in September 1948. My searches have revealed no convincing match.

Hutton, Andrew Michael (1916–1980) was a Guys anaesthetist who attended in December 1953 when hypothermia was discussed and February 1954 when ventricular fibrillation was the topic. He spoke from the floor on both occasions. Mike Hutton was one of the regular thoracic anaesthetists and had written with P. J. Helliwell and Ernest Rink on anaesthesia for operations on pulmonary stenosis.[227]
Q: Guys 1938; DA 1947; FFA RCS 1953

Jewsbury, Percy (1920–2008) attended the Club in May 1954 when he was a senior registrar in thoracic surgery at the Withington Hospital, Manchester. The following year he was appointed cardiothoracic surgeon at the Blackpool Victoria Hospital.
Q: MD Minnesota 1934; Manchester MB ChB 1944; FRCS 1950
http://livesonline.rcseng.ac.uk/biogs/E001032b.htm

Jordaan, Michael (-) attended regularly from September 1949 to April 1950. He was on Russell Brocks surgical firm at the time. Jordaan returned to South Africa and published on cardiac surgical subjects. Notably in 1954 he reported his first 100 operations for mitral stenosis, with three deaths and 93 patients improved, most of them greatly.[236-238]

Juvenelle, André A (?–?) was Chief Assistant-Surgeon, Head of Surgical Laboratories, Centre Chirurgical Marie-Lannelongue, Paris and attended the meeting in December 1953 when Donald Ross talked about hypothermia. Juvenelle was also working on the subject.[84]

Kauntze, Ralph (1911–2004) was an assistant physician when he attended meetings from December 1948 to February 1950. In 1956 he became physician to the cardiac department. Kauntze wrote with Maurice Campbell on cardiac topics.[239;240]
Q: Cambridge and St Georges 1937; MRCP 1939; MD 1946; FRCP 1950
http://munksroll.rcplondon.ac.uk/Biography/Details/5302

Kittle, Charles Frederick (1921–2015) was a thoracic surgeon in Kansas when a guest of the Club in May 1951. Dr Kittle worked in Kansas and then Chicago.

Q: Chicago 1945

http://www.athensnews.com/obituaries/dr-charles-frederick-kittle-md/article_9f4a3cc2-78f8-11e5-9e35-7f44c2f8dbc2.html

Knebel, R. attended four consecutive meetings from January to April 1951. (S)he was working in the Cardiac Department at Guys with a British Council Fellowship for German University Teachers and co-authored with Dennis Deuchar a big paper on systemic and pulmonary circulations in congenital heart disease.[78]

Lowe, James Brian (1917–1993) attended with a group of cardiologists in December 1949 when he was senior registrar in cardiology 1946 to 1950 at the Hammersmith, Brompton and National Heart Hospitals. Dr Lowe came from New Zealand to study medicine in Edinburgh. He was first assistant to Paul Wood at the Institute of Cardiology in 1951. He was acknowledged along with Wood and Brock for his contribution to a paper by Maurice McGregor on right ventricular hypertrophy.[241] In 1953 he was appointed cardiologist at Green Lane Hospital, Auckland and worked with the surgeon Rowan Nicks.

Q: Edinburgh 1940; MRCPE 1947; MRCP 1948; FRCPE 1957; FRCP 1967

http://munksroll.rcplondon.ac.uk/Biography/Details/2808

Macdonald, Ian (1921–2008) attended in April 1951. He was a physiologist in the medical school he wrote with Eddie Holling and Albert Venner about estimating blood oxygen.[235] Ian Macdonald was lecturer in physiology at Guys from 1948, reader from 1962, professor from 1967 and head of department from 1977. He taught me when I was a preclinical medical student at Guys 1965-7. He was prominent internationally in nutrition science.

Obituary *BMJ* 2009; 338 doi: https://doi.org/10.1136/bmj.b1436 (Published 07 April 2009)

McMillan, Ian Kenneth Ramsay (1922–1989) attended in July 1951 and February 1953 while he was a research fellow at the Royal College of Surgeons (1951–54). He had devised a means of filming the movement of

the heart valves. Mr McMillan was senior lecturer in the surgical unit at St Thomass before becoming consultant thoracic surgeon in Southampton in 1959. He published with colleagues working at St Thomas and Denis Melrose of the Hammersmith Hospital.[70;80;242;243]
Q: Cambridge and St Thomass 1948; FRCS 1956
http://livesonline.rcseng.ac.uk/biogs/E007497b.htm

Magidson, Oscar (1920–2003) attended with a group of cardiologists in December 1949 when he was registrar and senior registrar with Paul Wood at the National Heart Hospital.[244] Dr Magidson moved to Leeds then to California where he was a cardiologist, retiring in 1997.
Q: Leeds 1943; MRCP 1945; FRCP 1969
http://munksroll.rcplondon.ac.uk/Biography/Details/5117

Matthews, Michael Bernard (1920–2015) was probably a medical registrar when he attended the club with Ian McMillan in July 1951. He was one of a group including Richard Gorlin, researching and publishing together at St Thomass.[245] Dr Matthews was later a physician in Edinburgh.
Q: Cambridge and St Thomass 1944; MRCP 1946; MD 1954 FRCP Edinburgh 1959, FRCP 1966.
http://munksroll.rcplondon.ac.uk/Biography/Details/7101

McArdle, Brian (1911–2002) was at the Guys Clinical Research Unit and attended a Club meeting in July 1948 with Reginald Waterfield to discuss thrombosis and embolus associated with cyanotic heart disease. McArdle worked for the MRC at the National Hospital, Queen Square and in 1947 returned to Guys Clinical Research Unit. In 1951 he described the syndrome that bears his name[246] and published with David Verel on ischaemic muscle work.[247] There was an eminent elder brother John Michael Francis McArdle, a neurologist. The Club Minutes almost certainly refer to Brian McArdle.
Q: Guys 1933; MRCP 1936; MD 1937; FRCP 1960
http://munksroll.rcplondon.ac.uk/Biography/Details/5820

McGregor, Maurice (?–?) was working with Paul Wood as a registrar at the National Heart Hospital when he attended the meeting in December 1949 with a group of cardiologists.

McGregor acknowledged help from James Lowe in his publications on cardiac topics and co-authored with Paul Wood and Oscar Magidson.[248] Dr McGregor returned to Witwatersrand University Medical School and Johannesberg Hospital and in 1957 he went to the Department of Cardiology at Montreal Childrens Hospital.

Q: 1942 Witwatersrand; MD 1947; MRCP 1948

https://muhc.ca/patients/article/dr-maurice-mcgregor

McLaren, Lyall Robertson (1917–1980) attended three meetings in a row in April to June 1949 while doing his middle grade surgical training. McLaren went on to be a plastic surgeon in Manchester.

Q: Cambridge and Guys 1941; FRCS 1950.

Obituaries *The Lancet* 17 and *BMJ* 24 January 1981.

http://livesonline.rcseng.ac.uk/biogs/E006742b.htm

Milstein, Benjamin Bethel (1918–2013) spoke occasionally in meetings from November 1952 to December 1955 when he was Russell Brocks senior registrar. He presented data to the Club on ventricular fibrillation and vied with Ross on the best route for direct needle puncture to the left atrium (December 1955). He wrote with other Club members.[75;98;105;213;249-251] Ben Milstein was appointed as thoracic surgeon to the Brook Hospital, Greenwich and in 1957 to Papworth Hospital which he built up to be one of the most prestigious units in England. He was editor of *Thorax* from 1978.

Q: UCL 1942; FRCS 1947.

http://livesonline.rcseng.ac.uk/biogs/E004089b.htm

Neill, Catherine Annie (1921–2006) was a registrar at Queen Elizabeth Hospital for Children (QEH) in London when she attended the last recorded meeting of the Club in March 1956. She spoke on atrial septal defect. She had been working with Maurice Campbell in analysing the natural history of congenital heart disease.[108] Neill took the Diploma in Child Health in 1946. Her work at the QEH included admitting blue babies to bleed those with polycythaemic crises. She was influenced by a lecture in 1947 during Alfred Blalocks visit. Later she travelled to Canada and then to Johns Hopkins,

The Heart Club

extending her stay with Helen Taussig to three years. She returned to QEH as a consultant in 1954 but returned to Johns Hopkins after two years where she made her career.

Q: Royal Free Hospital 1944; DCH 1946; MD 1947; MRCP 1947; FRCP 1970

http://munksroll.rcplondon.ac.uk/Biography/Details/5609

Nicks, George Rowan (1913–2011) was a guest of the Club in January 1952 when came from New Zealand to study and visited in Europe and America. George Nicks was from Dunedin and had trained at the Brompton. He was appointed as surgeon in 1947 at Green Lane Hospital, Auckland, New Zealand where he worked with James Lowe. In 1952 he had study leave to visit John Kirklin at the Mayo Clinic, Alfred Blalock at Johns Hopkins and Russell Brock. He later moved to Sydney.

Q: 1937, FRCS Edinburgh 1942, FRACS 1948, ChM 1951

http://livesonline.rcseng.ac.uk/biogs/E001561b.htm

O'Connell, Thomas Columba James Bob (1906–1985) was a thoracic surgeon at St. Vincents Hospital, Dublin who visited in April 1949. OConnell studied in Berlin with Ferdinand Sauerbruch in 1933. In 1937–38 he worked with Arthur Tudor Edwards, Clement Price Thomas and Russell Brock at the Brompton. In 1945 he helped launch the Irish Society of Thoracic Surgeons. He reported the first ligation of a patent ductus arteriosus in Ireland in 1946, and a further series was reviewed in 1948. These may have been unpublished presentations. He was apparently notorious for advertising his firsts in the Dublin newspapers rather than reporting them in the medical literature. He devised a new technique for surgery of coarctation[252] and reported a successful emergency operation for mitral stenosis in the early stages of labour.[253]

Q: University College Dublin 1930; MD MCh; FRCSI 1962

Obituary *Irish Journal of Medical Science* September 1986, Volume 155, Issue 9, 311–316

O'Neill, Thomas J (?–?) attended at the same time as Denton Cooley in September 1950 and spoke on his experience with the surgery of mitral stenosis. ONeill was one of the team in Philadelphia where Charles Bailey had first success with mitral valve operation in 1948 along with Dwight Harken and Russell Brock.[64;65] In 1956 ONeill held surgical posts in several hospitals in Philadelphia.

Reinhold, John Drake Lucas (1922/3–1957) was a senior registrar in paediatrics at St Marys Hospital who presented phonocardiography records in aortic stenosis to the Club in December 1955, talked about septal defects in January 1956 and spoke on the heart sounds and ECG in atrial septal defect at the final meeting in March 1956. Dr Reinhold was appointed House Officer at Guys in May 1945. Later he was research registrar at the Canadian Red Cross Memorial Hospital in Taplow publishing regularly. He was appointed assistant professor in Denver Colorado in 1957 but was killed in a car crash before taking up his post, and before the publication of his last paper from Guys and Great Ormond Street Hospitals.[109]
Q: Oxford and Guys 1945; MRCP 1947; DCH 1951
Obituary: Lancet July 27 1957 P.199.

Rienhoff, William F. was a surgeon at Johns Hopkins. If it was Rienhoff (which seems likely although the name is spelt Rheinhoff in the Minutes) the only mention of him attending the Club was in February 1956. The Hopkins surgeon Bill Rienhoff was an exchange visitor to Guys for four weeks around September 1948. In a letter to Alfred Blalock during this time he wrote with great enthusiasm and described operating for Brock at the Brompton.[*]
Q: Johns Hopkins

Reynolds, Geoffrey Lewis Leslie (1915–present) was a regular attender from December 1948 to October 1951. It was agreed in November 1948 that as registrar in the cardiology department he was *ex officio* eligible for membership. He made continuous records of the ECG during angiocardiography[51] and presented work on this in July 1951 prompted by three deaths following this investigation. He published a series of papers with other members of the Club.[68;182;223;254-258] By 1958 Dr Reynolds was medical officer at Highlands School, Eldoret, Kenya but I could find no subsequent trace of him.
Q: Oxford and Guys 1940

---

[*] Letter in the Rienhoff collected papers in the Alan Mason Chesney Archives, Johns Hopkins

Rink, Ernest Herrmann (1903–1959) was anaesthetist for Russell Brocks first successful pulmonary valvotomy and other early heart operations and was a regular attender from the start of the Club until October 1951. In July 1948, he commented on the optimum positioning of the patient for mitral valve surgery in preparation for the start of operations on mitral stenosis and discussed the monitoring during cardiac surgery. He wrote about anaesthesia for cardiac surgery in Guys Hospital Reports and in the Annals of the Royal College of Surgeons.[227;259]
Q: Oxford and Guys 1930; DA 1935; FFA RCS 1948

Ross, Donald Nixon (1922–2014) spoke at Club meetings in December 1953 and December 1955. He was working at the time in the animal laboratory studying blood stream cooling as a means to reduce the blood flow and to thus extend circulatory arrest to make open heart surgery possible.[81;82;83] Donald Ross was born in South Africa and came to England to train with Ronald Belsey in Bristol. In 1953 he was appointed cardiovascular research fellow at Guys. The following year he became Russell Brocks senior registrar and in 1958 Brocks consultant colleague. Donald Ross went on to become the pre-eminent British heart surgeon and was deservedly internationally famous. He worked at Guys where I was his house surgeon in 1971. He later left Guys to work at The Middlesex Hospital where I was his consultant colleague in the 1980s. He worked also at the National Heart Hospital. He did the only three heart transplants in England in the 1970s. After the moratorium he never returned to transplantation.
Q: Cape Town 1946; FRCS 1949
http://livesonline.rcseng.ac.uk/biogs/E005828b.htm

Scott, George Walter (1923–2007) was a Guys houseman when he attended the Club as Mr Scott in September and November 1950. In 1951 a Dr Scott attended and showed a P.M. specimen of mitral stenosis. This was probably him. Scott was later a Fulbright Scholar and spent a year at Johns Hopkins. He became a consultant chest physician at Guys Hospital and was a popular teacher when I was a clinical student at Guys 1967-1970.
Q: Guys 1949; MD 1952; MRCP 1953; FRCP 1968
http://munksroll.rcplondon.ac.uk/Biography/Details/5585

Tom Treasure

Shephard, Roy Jesse (1929–present) was medically qualified and studying for a PhD in physiology when he attended the Club in February and March 1954 at meetings to discuss ventricular fibrillation and pulmonary blood flow. He was working in the cardiac department and published a series of papers in 1954 to 1956 in various journals.[85-97] He thanked Maurice Campbell and the surgeons whose patients he studied. This work contributed to his PhD thesis. Shephard went to Cincinnati and then Toronto and went on to make contributions in exercise physiology and medicine.[260;261]
Q Guys 1952; PhD 1954; MD 1960
http://injuryprevention.bmj.com/content/11/5/293.1.full

Schrire, Velva (1916-1972) was senior registrar at the National Heart Hospital (1949-50) when a guest of the Club in December 1949. Dr Schrire returned to Cape Town where he had qualified. He went on to be the director of the Cardiac Clinic in Groote Schuur. His publications echoed the themes of the Club.[262] He co-authored with Christiaan Barnard, *The Surgery of the Common Congenital Cardiac Malformations,* 1968.
Q: Cape Town 1941; MRCP 1950; FRCP 1962
http://munksroll.rcplondon.ac.uk/Biography/Details/3956

Sokolow, Maurice (1913?–2002) was an American cardiologist who attended in May 1954 when he was head of the hypertension section at San Francisco General Hospital Medical Center. He joined a discussion on ventricular pressures.
Q: MD UCSF 1936
https://www.ucsf.edu/news/2002/09/4854/maurice-sokolow-md
http://senate.universityofcalifornia.edu/_files/inmemoriam/html/MauriceSokolow. htm

Somerville, Walter (1913–2005) was an assistant to Paul Wood when he attended with him and other cardiologists as guests of the Club in December 1949. He qualified at the Mater Hospital in Dublin and was working in London when war was declared. He served in WW2, demobilised with the rank of lieutenant colonel and studied for two years largely in Boston where he met many American doctors who became lifelong friends. On return to London he became assistant to Paul Wood. He was appointed consultant

The Heart Club

cardiologist at Harefield Hospital in 1952 and at the Middlesex Hospital in 1954 where he worked with Thomas Holmes Sellors.

Q: University College Dublin 1937; MD 1940; FRCP 1957; CBE 1982.

http://munksroll.rcplondon.ac.uk/Biography/Details/5465

Soothill, Edward Farrar (1923–1961) was Russell Brocks houseman when he attended the Club from November 1948 to November 1949. Soothill trained in surgery in Norwich and went to Australia in 1961 where he was hit by a car and killed soon after disembarking from the ship.

Q: Cambridge and Guys 1948; FRCS 1955; MCh 1960

http://livesonline.rcseng.ac.uk/biogs/E005564b.htm

Starkey, George (1917–2000) attended the Club from October 51 to March 1952 during which time he was a trainee with Russell Brock. With Benjamin Milstein he wrote up a case of death after angiocardiography.[249] Starkey had trained in surgery at Bellevue and other hospitals in New York City. When he returned to America he practised cardiothoracic surgery in the Boston area.

Q: Harvard

http://articles.courant.com/2000-02-13/
news/0002111563_1_harvard-medical-school-surgery-boston-city-hospital

Stevens. A Dr Stevens attended in April 1949 but has not been identified and was possibly junior staff.

Suzman, Samuel Sappy (?–?) was a clinical assistant in the cardiography department and a regular attender and was at the first and the last meeting. He published with Campbell and others.[108;175;263] Dr Suzman had an honorary appointment in Sevenoaks Hospital.

Q: Guys 1923; MRCP1931

Trounce, John Reginald (1920–2007) attended from April 1950 to April 1951 probably when he was clinically attached to the cardiac department, publishing papers with Charles Baker, Maurice Campbell and Geoffrey Reynolds.[69;116;121;182;264] John Trounce co-authored the Residents Play in April 1948 and he was house physician to Boland and Baker from November 1948. He went on to work at the Brompton Hospital and the National Heart Hospital before going back to Guys. He was a research fellow at Johns

Hopkins 1960– 1961. He came back with the determination to start three developments at Guys: set up an oncology clinic, start a renal dialysis unit, and teach clinical pharmacology to medical students as a separate subject. He achieved all three.

Q: Guys 1943; MRCP 1944; MD 1946; FRCP 1964

http://munksroll.rcplondon.ac.uk/Biography/Details/5590

Van't Hoff, Walter (1924–2002) was a houseman at Guys and the Brompton when he attended in January and April 1951. He became a consultant endocrinologist in North Staffordshire.

Q: Cambridge 1946; MRCP 1952; FRCP 1971

http://munksroll.rcplondon.ac.uk/Biography/Details/5163

Venner, Albert (?–?) attended the Club from March 1952 to May 1954 while a medical research fellow at Guys and published prolifically. [100;101;205;235] He went to Canada and worked in Edmonton, Alberta.

Q: KCL and Charing Cross 1942; MRCP 1947; MD 1950.

Verel, David (1919–2009) was a research fellow in the Guys Clinical Research Unit when he attended in February 1951 and October 1951, the year he became a lecturer in medicine at the London Hospital. He presented measurements of intra-arterial pressure during surgery for mitral stenosis. He wrote with members of the Club on various topics related to the cardiovascular system and circulation. [247;265-270] He became a consultant cardiologist in Sheffield in1957.

Q: Cambridge and the London 1943; MRCP 1945; MD 1948; FRCP 1967

http://munksroll.rcplondon.ac.uk/Biography/Details/6285

Waterfield, Reginald Lawson (1900–1986) was haematologist to Guys Hospital when he attended in July 1948 and with Brian McArdle joined discussion on blood viscosity and thrombosis. Reggie Lawson had been a House Physician at Guys and spent 1927-1929 as lecturer and assistant physician at Johns Hopkins. In WW2 he worked with blood transfusion services. In 1949 he had poliomyelitis which left him paraplegic, despite which he continued to work.

Q: Guys 1925; MRCP 1933; FRCP 1955

http://munksroll.rcplondon.ac.uk/Biography/Details/4640

The Heart Club

Whillis, James (1900–1955) Professor of Anatomy at Guys and editor of *Gray's Anatomy* and co-author with Gerald Channell.[192;193] There is no record that he attended the Club but he may well have been present in January 1949 when Rupert Willis gave a talk in his anatomy department, a venue which Rupert Willis had requested.
http://livesonline.rcseng.ac.uk/biogs/E005489b.htm

Whitaker, William (1919–2007) was a cardiologist training with Paul Wood at the National Heart Hospital when he attended the Club in December 1949. He went to the University of Sheffield as a senior lecturer in medicine. In 1956 he became a consultant physician and cardiologist in Leeds.
Q: Leeds 1943; MD 1946; MRCP 1948; FRCP 1963
http://munksroll.rcplondon.ac.uk/Biography/Details/5606

Willis, Rupert Allan (1898–1980), an Australian, was Collins Professor of Human and Comparative Pathology at the Hunterian Museum of the Royal College of Surgeons when he attended in January 1949. Willis gave a talk on the embryology of the heart in the Anatomy Department to which George Foxon contributed. Willis held a Rockefeller fellowship in 1933 and worked on embryology at the Buckstone Browne Research Farm, Downe, Kent, under Sir Arthur Keith. In 1948 was made director of pathology at the Royal Cancer Hospital, Fulham and in 1950 became professor of pathology at the University of Leeds.
Author of *The Borderland of Embryology and Pathology* (1958)[271]
Q: Melbourne 1922; MD 1929; DSc 1932
http://adb.anu.edu.au/biography/willis-rupert-allan-12039

Whytehead, Lawrence Layard (1914–2005) attended the club regularly from January 1949 to March 1951 while a senior registrar with Russell Brock. Whytehead had served in the RAF specialising in thoracic surgery during WW2. After training at Guys he became first assistant at the Brompton. He was the first recipient of the Evarts Graham memorial travelling fellowship established in 1951 and published basic science papers.[272;273] He published on pneumonectomy with Brock in 1955.[149] He was appointed at the Brook Hospital and Grove Park hospitals, London. In 1955 he emigrated to Canada.
Q: Oxford and Middlesex 1938; FRCS 1947
http://livesonline.rcseng.ac.uk/biogs/E000430b.htm

Wood, Paul Hamilton (1907–1962) was cardiologist to Brompton Hospital when he visited in December 1949 and with him was Walter Somerville and their trainees and fellows. By this time Wood was a prominent figure in cardiology. He came from Australia and by 1949 he had held several senior posts in London. In 1950 he was made director of the Institute of Cardiology at the National Heart Hospital. Paul Wood was co-author on the paper reporting the 100 mitral valvotomies[118] and according to McMichael he closed his 1954 Strickland Goodall Lectures by saying The trouble with mitral stenosis is mitral stenosis! thus conclusively debunking the Mackenzie-Lewis conviction that the trouble in mitral stenosis was the myocardium.[45] He died of myocardial infarction aged 55.
Q: Melbourne 1931; MRCP 1933; MD 1940; FRCP 1940
http://munksroll.rcplondon.ac.uk/Biography/Details/4869

Woods, Arnold Winkelried William Belmont (1915–1986) was senior registrar at the National Heart Hospital when he was one of the group of ten who attended by invitation the meeting in December 1949. He studied the ECGs of Campbells patients with congenital heart disease and published the results in the *BHJ* in 1952 .[274] He became consultant physician to Epsom District Hospital.
Q: Oxford 1940; MRCP 1943; MRCP 1943; FRCP 1965
http://munksroll.rcplondon.ac.uk/Biography/Details/4882

Zak, George Albert (1913-1984) worked in Guys Clinical Research Unit and was a regular attender of the Club from June 1948 until April 1951. According to Dennis Deuchar (Peacock Minutes March 1951) Dr Zak introduced the technique to the hospital November 1947 when he reviewed the results of 187 cardiac catheterisations done by the end of 1950. Zak wrote an appendix on cardiac catheterisation for the 1948 paper on the first 50 Blalock shunts. [115] He published with Eddie Holling and Dennis Deuchar.[204;231] George Zak qualified in Vienna in 1937 and but was on the British Medical Register from July 1941 presumably having left Austria around the start of WW2. He later moved to New York University where he was a Fellow in Physiology 1951–53, Instructor in Medicine 1953–61, Assistant Professor of Clinical Medicine 1961–68 and Associate Professor from 1968 to his death in 1984. His clinical positions were at Bellevue. He continued to publish on physiology and clinical science.[275;276]
Q: Vienna 1937

Author networks

By a process of electronic and paper searching in PubMed, Index Medicus and the contents of *Guy's Hospital Reports* it was not difficult to amass a large list of citations. Many of the Club members published prolifically. A consistent pattern was that research work presented in the Peacock Club would appear not long after in print. Work in progress or recently completed research by trainees, and fellows in the course of writing their MD, MS or PhD theses was published in long form in *Guy's Hospital Reports (GHR)* of which Russell Brock was the editor at the time. Working with John Kirklin in the University of Alabama in Birmingham in 1981 I had found *GHR* on the library shelves; the journal had a long reach. It was influential in this era. For example, in the course of research with John Kirklin on hypothermic circulatory arrest, I used the oxygen consumption data obtained in experiments in Guys by Donald Ross[81;82;152] in my own research on hypothermia.[277-279] Donald Ross had published it in detail in *Guy's Hospital Reports*.

A distillation of the research first published in *GHR* might later be sent to the *British Heart Journal* where Maurice Campbell was editor from 1938 to 1958. It cant escape notice that there might have been an inside track to publication in both journals. However, the work of Peacock Club members was also published in leading national and international journals.

As an illustrative exercise I have performed an author network analysis to get an impression of the collaborations. The first version using the authors only showed many interconnections. We are now accustomed to papers with multiple authors. Because of many one and two author papers, the network method underestimated the extent of collaborations within the Club and the clinical team. I repeated the exercise including those who were acknowledged for what appeared to be a substantial contribution to the work. A number of additional names appear in the second network, perhaps giving a more representative idea of the extent of the teamwork. The network display gives an impression of the dominant influence of Campbell and Brock within the group but they were there throughout the time of the Club while most of the younger members were passing through. Where these many young doctors came from, and where they ended up, as shown in the Biographical Notes (List 1) is of interesting.

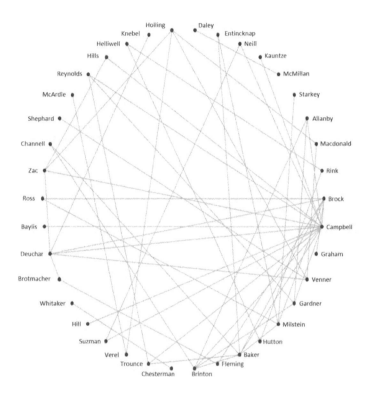

Co-author network of Peacock Club publications.

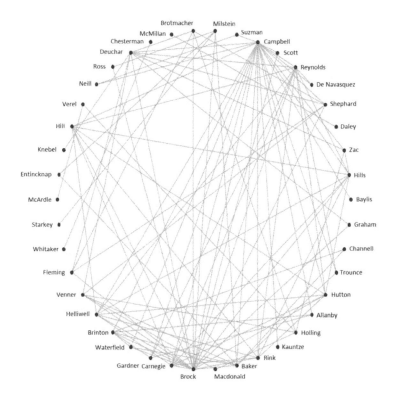

Author and acknowledgement network.

Biographical Notes: List 2

This list includes those whose work was discussed at the Peacock Club but who were not among known attendees, and others whose names feature in the book. Many in this list have copious biographical records. Where there is a reliable internet source it is provided. Qualifications are only given for British entries. Other countries tend to have a generic MD but British doctors have many letters after their names which are informative.

Atkins, Hedley John Barnard (1904–1983) was educated at Trinity College, Oxford and Guys. Before the war all his appointments had been at Guys. In 1942 he went to North Africa with the RAMC and subsequently served in Italy and was demobilised with the rank of Lieutenant-Colonel. He was appointed the first director of the Guys department of surgery in 1947. He is best known for his commitment to breast surgery[280-286] but at the time of the Club he was engaged in a series of thoracolumbar sympathectomy operations (Smithwicks operation) to treat hypertension. This from information from the Guys Hospital Operating theatre books studied in the London Metropolitan Archive. Atkins admired the training relationship between Alfred Blalock and Henry Bahnson and in a long handwritten letter on 1st November 1947 (addressed to My dear Al) he regarded the approach to surgical training at Johns Hopkins as something to strive for at Guys. This I found in documents which I studied in the Alan Mason Chesney Archives of the Johns Hopkins Medical Institutions. Hedley Atkins was appointed the first professor of surgery at Guys in 1961.
Q: MB BCh 1932; FRCS 1934; KBE 1967.
http://livesonline.rcseng.ac.uk/biogs/E000236b.htm

Bailey, Charles Philamore (1910–1993) was a lecturer at Hahnemann University Hospital and a surgeon at Episcopal Hospital Philadelphia. In 1948 he reported four operations on mitral stenosis from November 1945

using a punch or knife to perform what he called commissurotomy. He had his first survivor at his 4th attempt on 10th June 1948.[48] Bailey was made professor and head of thoracic surgery at Hahnemann, a post he held for 10 years (1948–58). Bailey appears in the Minutes (February 1950) when In connexion with the work on Mitral stenosis, Russell Brock particularly mentioned the work of Bailey, Glover & ONeill in Philadelphia.[64;65;66] ONeill came to the Peacock Club in September 1950.
http://onlinelibrary.wiley.com/doi/10.1002/clc.4960280413/pdf

Bahnson, Henry (Hank) (1920–2003) came to Guys as Blalocks assistant in 1947 where he was nicknamed Haemostasis Henry by the Guys residents, according to Ken Citron who was a medical student on Brocks firm at the time. Bahnson named his second son Blalock. Hank Bahnson remained at Johns Hopkins until 1963 when he became professor and chairman of surgery at the University of Pittsburgh School of Medicine where he stayed until 1987.
https://www.ncbi.nlm.nih.gov/pmc/articles/PMC1514482/

Bedford, Davis Evan (1898–1978) was an international authority on cardiology in the 1930s and 1940s. He was a Middlesex Hospital graduate and served briefly in WW1 and returning to his medical school to qualify in 1921. Evan Bedford worked with John Parkinson at the London Hospital and in 1926 was appointed assistant physician to The Middlesex Hospital and in 1933 physician to outpatients at the National Heart Hospital. Walter Somerville wrote of Evan Bedford He felt a special kinship in the early days of cardiac surgery with Holmes Sellors and Brock, and spent many hours in the operating theatre.
Q: MB BS London 1921; MD 1925; FRCP 1931; CBE 1963.
http://munksroll.rcplondon.ac.uk/Biography/Details/331

Beck, Claude Schaeffer (1894–1971) was professor of cardiovascular surgery (1952–65) at Western Reserve University Medical School and is cited twice in the Minutes in connection with work in the revascularisation of the heart (February 1950) and that he had given up his anastomosis of aorta and coronary sinus. (December 1954). In the 1920s he did experimental work with Cutler related to surgery for mitral stenosis[287] and was co-author on the final report[39] which effectively called a moratorium.[288] He wrote on defibrillation

in 1941[289] and performed the first successful cardiac defibrillation in a human in 1947 following work with Carl Wiggers and George Crile.
http://artsci.case.edu/dittrick/online-exhibits/explore-the-artifacts/claude-beck-defibrillation-and-cpr/

Beechar, Henry Knowles (1904–1976) was from 1941 Henry Isaiah Dorr Professor of Anaesthesia Research at Harvard Medical School. He appears in the Minutes along with John Heysham Gibbon in connection with ventilation studies (October 1951).
https://en.wikipedia.org/wiki/Henry_K._Beecher

Bing, Richard John (1909–2010), was a German refugee who became a leading cardiologist in the USA. He was publishing experimental work with right heart catheterisation at Johns Hopkins from 1947.[52-55] Maurice Campbell witnessed his work during his visit to Johns Hopkins in 1948 and Russell Brock met him in 1949. A little later Bing was able to sample coronary sinus blood during cardiac catheterisation and applied the Fick principle to study myocardial oxygen consumption.[201] His name and references to his work appear several times in the Minutes.
https://en.wikipedia.org/wiki/Richard_Bing

Bishop, Peter Maxwell Farrow (1904–1979) was notable in this history for running the Emergency Medical Service living in the Wardens House at Guys and firefighting as necessary. He was prominent in gynaecological endocrinology.
Q Oxford 1929; DM 1943; MRCP 1951; FRCP 1957; FRCOG 1967
http://munksroll.rcplondon.ac.uk/Biography/Details/409

Björk, Viking Olov (1918–2009) was a surgeon at Sabbatsberg Hospital (Stockholm), working with Clarence Crafoord when his operation for atrial septal defect was favourably mentioned by Russell Brock in November 1954. Björk had been a registrar at the Brompton Hospital where he worked with Arthur Tudor Edwards and Clement Price. He became head of cardiovascular surgery at Uppsala University (1958–66).
https://www.ncbi.nlm.nih.gov/pmc/articles/PMC2720303/

The Heart Club

Blalock, Alfred (1899–1964) was chief of surgery at the Johns Hopkins Hospital and professor and director of the department of surgery of the medical school when in 1944 he performed the first blue baby operation, a subclavian to pulmonary artery anastomosis, on a 15-month-old child.[18] Although the baby died a few months later, Blalock eventually carried out his operation on thousands of children. Blalock carried out nine or ten of his subclavian pulmonary artery anastomosis operations to introduce the procedure at Guys Hospital in September 1947.[290]
https://en.wikipedia.org/wiki/Alfred_Blalock

Boland, Edward Rowan Bo (1898–1972) was a physician at Guys Hospital, Dean of the Medical School (1945–65) and Dean of the Faculty of Medicine, University of London (1948–52) and so played an important role in implementing post war changes in the organisation of medical education at Guys. He set up the exchange scheme with his opposite number at Johns Hopkins, Alan Mason Chesney. The East Wing of Guys destroyed by WW2 bombing was named after Boland when it was rebuilt.
Q: MRCS LRCP1923; FRCP 1934; Kt 1964.
http://munksroll.rcplondon.ac.uk/Biography/Details/458

Chesney, Alan Mason was an infectious disease specialist and dean of the Johns Hopkins School of Medicine. The schools of medicine, nursing, and public health archive their collective history in the Alan Mason Chesney Medical Archives. I am grateful to its archivists for access to their collection in February 2017 in the course of research for this book.

Cournand, André Frédéric (1895–1988), was born in Paris, and was a professor at the Columbia University College of Physicians and Surgeons and worked at Bellevue Hospital in New York City. From there with Dickinson Richards he published a series of studies in the 1940s that established use of cardiac catheterization as a routine procedure, employing it to measure pressure and oxygen content, including using contrast media for x-ray images.[56] His name appears four times in the Minutes.
http://onlinelibrary.wiley.com/doi/10.1002/clc.4960090207/pdf

Crafoord, Clarence (1899–1984), performed the first successful repair of coarctation of the aorta in October 1944[23] and he was prominent in the

reported meetings around the time the Club was being formed.[20;21;23;24;291-293] He was a surgeon at Sabbatsberg Hospital in Stockholm and had studied briefly in the USA just before WW2. He became professor of thoracic surgery at the Karolinska Institute, Stockholm 1948–66. He was well known to surgeons throughout the world for surgery of coarctation. His work was mentioned twice in the Minutes (November 1953, February 1955).
http://www.annalsthoracicsurgery.org/article/S0003-4975(08)02076-6/fulltext

Cutler, Elliot Carr (1888–1947) in the 1920s did a series of operations for mitral stenosis.[39;44;287] After an initial survivor he had a run of deaths leading to a final report[39] and a voluntary moratorium.[288] He went on to become Surgeon-in-Chief at Peter Bent Brigham Hospital from 1932 to 1947. During WW2 he rose to be Brigadier General in the U.S. Army Medical Corps. He was opposed to specialist services but was probably out manoeuvred by Paul Hawley and Tudor Edwards[13] allowing Dwight Harken the opportunity to demonstrate that the chambers of the heart could be instrumented without fatal consequences.[14]
http://ech.case.edu/cgi/article.pl?id=CEC1
https://en.wikipedia.org/wiki/Elliott_Cutler

Ebstein, Wihelm (1836–1912) was a German physician. Describe in 1866 the anomaly which bears his name and which occurred several times in the discussion of cases at the Peacock Club.
https://www.ncbi.nlm.nih.gov/pubmed/11675224

Edwards, Arthur Tudor (1890–1946) was a key figure in the history of thoracic surgery who died before the Club was formed. He was widely admired for his surgical skill and was an inspiration and role model for those who worked with him in the 1930s including Russell Brock and others who developed cardiac surgery after 1945. Trained at The Middlesex Hospital and commissioned in the RAMC in 1914, he became assistant surgeon to the Brompton Hospital where he developed the surgery of the thorax into a modern speciality. In 1936 he became first Director of the Department of Thoracic Surgery at the London Hospital. In 1939–45 he was a civilian consultant with the Royal Air Force and adviser for thoracic casualties to the Ministry of Health.
Q: Cambridge and the Middlesex 1913: MRCS 1915; FRCS 1915.
http://livesonline.rcseng.ac.uk/biogs/E004015b.htm

Fallot, Étienne-Louis Arthur (1850–1911) was made Professor of Hygiene and Legal Medicine in Marseille in 1888, the year he described the four anatomical characteristics that constitute the Tetralogy of Fallot, one of the congenital heart defects responsible for blue babies. Campbell regarded Peacocks description in 1858, 30 years before, as having a better claim for an eponym so while he did not propose changing the name of the condition he wanted to name the club after Peacock.[2]
https://en.wikipedia.org/wiki/Arthur_Fallot

Fick, Adolf Eugen (1829–1901) was a German-born physician and physiologist. He first studied mathematics and physics. In 1855 he described Ficks law of diffusion and in 1870 measured cardiac output by what is known as the Fick principle. See the Glossary for further mention.
https://en.wikipedia.org/wiki/Adolf_Eugen_Fick

Gibbon, John Heysham (1903-1973) became director of surgical research at the Jefferson Medical College in 1946. He had worked for many years on pulmonary physiology with the ambition of producing a heart lung machine. Gibbon is mentioned in the Minutes along with Henry K. Beecher in connection with ventilation studies (October 1951) and in March 1955 when Russell Brock described Gibbons heart lung machine as expensive and complicated.
http://circ.ahajournals.org/content/107/17/2168

Graham, Evarts Ambrose (1883–1957) was Bixby Professor of Surgery at Washington University in St. Louis. Widely famous as a thoracic surgeon between the wars his clinic was visited by European surgeons including Russell Brock who was there in 1930. He was a moderniser who sought to reform surgery on academic lines. He was much admired in Britain as well as at home and was awarded the Lister Medal of the Royal College of Surgeons in 1942.
http://www.nasonline.org/publications/biographical-memoirs/memoir-pdfs/graham-evarts.pdf

Grant, Ronald Thomson (1892–1989) was appointed first director of the MRC department of clinical research at Guys Hospital in 1934 where he remained, except for wartime, until 1957. Apparently he didnt get on well

with clinicians but a number of researchers from his unit, such as his more accommodating colleague Eddie Holling, played an important part in the Peacock Club. He enlisted in WW1 but invalidity prevented him serving and he qualified in 1915. He had a clinical post in Glasgow in 1919 and then obtained a research post in Sir Thomas Lewis MRC funded cardiographic department at University College Hospital, London, where he studied soldiers heart.
Q: MB ChB 1915; MD 1922; FRS 1934; FRCP 1951; OBE 1947
http://munksroll.rcplondon.ac.uk/Biography/Details/1859.

Gross, Robert Edward (1905–1988) was professor of child surgery at Harvard Medical School and the surgeon-in-chief at the Childrens Hospital in Boston (1947–66). In 1938 he successfully closed a patent ductus arteriosus in a seven-year-old girl and many subsequent cases.[294] Shortly afterwards he began experimental animal work on correcting coarctation of the aorta which he undertook on patients shortly after the war. In February 1950 in the Peacock Club, Russell Brock singled out the high standard of Grosss work.
https://www.nap.edu/read/4961/chapter/8

Glover, Robert P. (?–2006) was assistant clinical professor of surgery at the University of Pennsylvania School of Medicine and one of the team, along with Thomas J. E. ONeill* when Charles P. Bailey started operating on mitral stenosis in the 1940s.[48;64;66]

Harken, Dwight Emary (1910–1993) was chief of thoracic surgery at Peter Bent Brigham Hospital (1948-1970) As Captain Dwight Harken of the US Army in Europe, working at the 160th US General Hospital near Cirencester, UK, he performed a series of 134 operations for removal of shrapnel pieces and other missiles in and around the heart.[14] He operated on mitral stenosis by what he called valvuloplasty in 1947 and had his first survivor on 16th June 1948.[49]
https://en.wikipedia.org/wiki/Dwight_Harken

Hawley, Paul Ramsey (1891–1965) was Command Surgeon of the European Theater of Operations, US Army from January 1942 to May 1945. His

---

* See ONeill in biographies of the Peacock Club attendees.

The Heart Club

expertise was in public health and administration but according to Harkens biographer, Hawley gave Dwight Harken the opportunity to lead a specialist thoracic service in Cirencester UK in 1944.[14]
https://en.wikipedia.org/wiki/Paul_Ramsey_Hawley

Hill, Archibald Vivian (1886–1977), known as A. V. Hill, was a Fellow of the Royal Society (FRS) from 1918. From 1923 until his retirement in 1951 he was professor of physiology at University College, London. He shared the 1922 Nobel Prize in Physiology and Medicine for studies of heat production during muscle activity. He was noted in the Minutes of April 1949 in connection with the Bing test and blood gas analysis.
https://www.nobelprize.org/nobel_prizes/medicine/laureates/1922/hill-bio.html

Hollman, Arthur (1923–2013) was cardiologist at University College Hospital. He was a keen medical historian and Thomas Lewis biographer.[295] He worked at Taplow, held research posts in Toronto and Montreal in 1951 and 1952, and was Paul Woods assistant at the National Heart Hospital. He was senior registrar at the Royal Postgraduate Medical School and in 1959 was a member of the team that went to Moscow with the Melrose heart–lung machine.
Q 1946 UCL; MRCP 1947; MD 1950; FRCP1967
http://munksroll.rcplondon.ac.uk/Biography/Details/6935

Hufnagel, Charles A (1916–1989) was director of the surgical research laboratory and professor of surgery at Georgetown University, Washington DC. In 1952 he implanted a plastic non-return valve in the aorta for valvular incompetence.[296] The Hufnagel valve was implanted in several hundred more patients. It was noted at three Club meetings. In December 1954 Russell Brock remarked that it was dangerous.
https://en.wikipedia.org/wiki/Charles_A._Hufnagel

Hunter, William (1718–1783), the man-midwife and anatomist who in 1783 published post mortem findings of three cases showing marked cardiac abnormalities one of which was later identified as Fallots Tetralogy. This publication was discussed at a meeting of the Club (June 1949) together with the work of Thomas Bevill Peacock who had cited it. Thus it is clear that the

Hunter referred to in the Minutes was William and not his brother John who is said to have described a case later designated Fallots in an unpublished case book (CJL).[297]

https://www.ncbi.nlm.nih.gov/pmc/articles/PMC1236820/pdf/brheartj00104-0001.pdf

Keith, Arthur (1866–1955) was a world-famous figure who published widely on anatomy and anthropology and was important to the Club for studies he made soon after 1908 when he became Curator of the Museum of the Royal College of Surgeons. This work provided insights into the embryological development of pulmonary stenosis (Minutes June 1949).

https://www.ncbi.nlm.nih.gov/pmc/articles/PMC479569/pdf/brheartj00389-0137.pdf

Lillehei, Clarence Walton (1918–1999) was professor at the department of surgery, University of Minnesota (1951–67). Walt Lillehei used cross circulation to enable open heart surgery for repair of ventricular septal defects.[298] His work was reported to the Club by Russell Brock (December 1954, March 1955).

https://en.wikipedia.org/wiki/C_Walton_Lillehei

Meckel, Johann Friedrich (1781–1833) was a German anatomist whose studies of congenital heart disease were discussed at the Club (April 1949) with those of William Hunter and Thomas Bevill Peacock who referred extensively to Meckel and especially to his doctoral thesis *De cordis conditionibus abnormibus* of 1802.

https://en.wikipedia.org/wiki/Johann_Friedrich_Meckel

Montgomery, Hugh (-) was chief of the peripheral vascular clinic, Edward B. Robinette Foundation, at the University of Pennsylvania Medical School and worked with Jack Gibbon. When Eddie Holling recounted to the Club in November 1953 the details of a trip to the USA he reported working with Montgomery on measuring the oxygen tension of muscle.

O'Shaughnessy, Laurence Frederick (1900–1940) was one of the small group of British thoracic surgeons contemplating cardiac surgery in the late 1930s when he was the first research scholar to be appointed at the Buckston Browne Farm, Downe, and thoracic surgeon to the British Legion

The Heart Club

Sanatorium, near Maidstone, Kent. He published on thoracic surgery, surgical shock and experimental studies. Apparently he wrote a lecture on the possibility of pulmonary valvotomy, but such a lecture has not been discovered.[13] Harkens biographer believed that it was discussed between Harken and Brock in Cirencester at the 160th US Army Hospital. OShaughnessy went to war in September 1939 and was killed during an air raid at Dunkirk.[299]

Q: MB BS Durham 1923; FRCS 1926; MD 1930.

http://livesonline.rcseng.ac.uk/biogs/E004406b.htm

Pate, J. W. (-) At the meeting in November 1953 Eddie Holling reported his trip to the USA and spoke of Sawyer and Pates work on the injury current in arterial grafts and its effects on Thrombosis. [300;301]

Peacock, Thomas Bevill (1812–1882) was a physician interested in heart disease who founded the London Chest Hospital then called the Victoria Park Hospital which opened in 1855. His book *On malformations, &c., of the human heart: with original cases* (1858) was based on clinical observations but more especially post mortems, observations of specimens and wide reading. One is on the cover of this book, and is an example of Fallots Tetralogy. Maurice Campbell proposed that the Club be called after Peacock and so it was.

http://munksroll.rcplondon.ac.uk/Biography/Details/3493

Peterson, Lysle (-) was professor of physiology in surgery, University of Pennsylvania School of Medicine when Eddie Holling recounted to the Club in November 1953 the details of a trip to the USA and reported working with Peterson on measurement of acceleration of blood along the aorta.

Pezzi, C. (-) is mentioned in the Minutes (February 1951) as an Italian who introduced the graphic term hilar dance – vigorous pulmonary artery pulsations due to increased blood flow, visible fluoroscopically. The information was provided by Maurice Campbell who knew Pezzis publication and cited it.[67]

Potts, Willis (1895–1963) was surgeon-in-chief at the Childrens Memorial Hospital Chicago. He devised a side to side anastomosis between the descending aorta and the left pulmonary artery as an alternative to Alfred

256

Blalocks subclavian pulmonary artery anastomosis to relieve the cyanosis due to pulmonary stenosis in a 21-month-old child.[302] He subsequently carried out one or other of the operations on a large number of cases. This work was noted the meetings in February 1950 and November 1953.
http://www.annalsthoracicsurgery.org/article/S0003-4975(10)62371-5/abstract

Richards, Dickinson Woodruff (1895–1973 was made professor of medicine at Columbia University in 1947. By this time he was carrying out the cardiac catheterisation studies with André Cournand cited at the Club.[56]
https://en.wikipedia.org/wiki/Dickinson_W._Richards

Samways, Daniel West (1857–1932) studied Physics in Cambridge and researched and published from Zurich. His subsequent clinical training was at Guys. He practiced for most of his summers in Menton, on the French Riviera principally caring for British patients with rheumatic heart disease or tuberculosis. Among many things he took an interest in mitral stenosis. He wrote letters to *The Lancet* and the *BMJ* on matters of the day and was quick to challenge ideas that seemed to him illogical or unfounded.
Q. Cambridge and Guys 1891; MD 1894; MRCP 1899

Sawyer, P. N. (-). At the meeting in November 1953 Holling reported his trip to the USA and spoke of Sawyer and Pates work on the injury current in arterial grafts and its effects on Thrombosis.[303]

Sellors, Thomas Holmes (1902–1987) was always referred to as Holmes Sellors or as Uncle Tom. He was named in the Peacock Minutes in March 1953 when the post mortem findings in a patient of his were presented. He was appointed to the staff of the London Chest Hospital in 1934. He was thoracic surgeon to The Middlesex Hospital where, as in the Peacock Club, close collaboration was developed between the surgeon and the cardiologists; in his case the physicians were Evan Bedford and later Walter Somerville. Holmes Sellors carried out the first successful relief of pulmonary stenosis by direct operation in 1947.[29]
Q: BM BCh Oxford 1926; FRCS 1930; Kt 1963.
http://livesonline.rcseng.ac.uk/biogs/E000237b.htm

The Heart Club

Somerville, Jane (1933-present) is a cardiologist who is celebrated for developing services for what she dubbed Grown Up Congenital Heart (GUCH) disease. She came to Guys as Jane Platnauer and was Russell Brocks house surgeon. She married Walter Somerville in 1957 and they have four children. She was involved in the care of two of the patients who tell their stories in the book. She was consultant cardiologist at the National Heart Hospital.
Q. Guys 1955; MRCP 1957; FRCP 1973

Souttar, Henry Sessions (1875–1964) was a surgeon at the London Hospital who on 16th May 1925 operated on a girl aged 15, inserted his index finger into the left atrium via the atrial appendage, and dilated the mitral valve.[36] She lived for seven years and is in the table of ten cases published by Cutler in his final report in 1929.[39] Souttar served in Belgium in WW1 and spent his surgical career at the London. At his funeral service the lesson was read by Russell Brock.
Q: Oxford 1906; FRCS 1909; CBE 1919; Kt 1949.
http://livesonline.rcseng.ac.uk/biogs/E005565b.htm

Starr, Isaac (1895–1989), a cardiologist, was Hartzell Professor of Research Therapeutics at the University of Pennsylvania School of Medicine (1933–61). When Eddie Holling recounted to the Club in November 1953 the details of a trip to the USA he reported working with Starr on ballistocardiography.[304]
https://en.wikipedia.org/wiki/Isaac_Starr

Sturridge, Marvin Francis (1926–2017) was a cardiothoracic surgeon at The Middlesex and the London Chest Hospitals. He was the surgeon who in 1979 operated on Geraldine West to repair her Fallots Tetralogy.
Q: The Middlesex 1952; FRCS 1958; MS 1965
https://livesonline.rcseng.ac.uk/biogs/E009313b.htm

Taussig, Helen Brooke (1898–1986) was chief of the paediatric department of Johns Hopkins Hospital (1930–1963). She was interested in correlating clinical symptoms with congenital heart abnormalities, a group of disorders then of only pathological interest. She developed her idea of a shunt operation with the surgeon Alfred Blalock who first carried it out in 1944.[18] It was then called the Blalock-Taussig shunt and is now referred to as the Blalock–Thomas–Taussig operation acknowledging Vivien Thomas who did

258

the development work in the dog and advised Blalock in the operating room for the initial cases.

https://cfmedicine.nlm.nih.gov/physicians/biography_316.html

Thomas, Clement Price (1893–1973) was a thoracic surgeon from the Tudor Edwards circle at the Brompton. He was appointed to Westminster Hospital in 1927. He invited Clarence Crafoord there to demonstrate his operation for coarctation of the aorta in 1946. He was also surgeon to the Brompton. Q: Cardiff Medical School and the Westminster Hospital Medical 1921: FRCS 1923.

http://livesonline.rcseng.ac.uk/biogs/E006026b.htm

Thomas, Vivien Theodore (1910–1985) worked for Alfred Blalock as his surgical technician. He was a skilled operator in the dog lab and under Dr Blalocks direction tried to create a model of central cyanosis. Helen Taussig had noted that children with Fallots Tetralogy and a patent ductus fared better and proposed that they worked out how to copy this circulation in the laboratory. Diverting the subclavian artery to make an end to side anastomosis to the pulmonary artery proved to be the solution. When Blalock did his first few operations of this type he had Vivien Thomas stand close behind him to advise him on technical details. Thomas was never formally recognised at the time but in 1976 received an honorary doctorate from Johns Hopkins.

https://en.wikipedia.org/wiki/Vivien_Thomas

Tubbs, Oswald Sydney (1908–1993) was one of the Tudor Edwards circle who ligated an infected ductus arteriosus in 1939 and in 1943 he reported the closure of nine infected ducts.[22] Tubbs had tuberculosis as a young man and Russell Brock resected a lobe of his lung. He held consultant posts at St Bartholomews and was surgeon to the Brompton Hospital. Q: Cambridge and St Bartholomews 1932; FRCS 1935.

http://livesonline.rcseng.ac.uk/biogs/E008384b.htm

The Heart Club

Wiggers, Carl John (1883–1963), was professor of physiology from 1918-1953 at Western Reserve University School of Medicine where he and his many students were world authorities on cardiac physiology. His studies of the pulse tracings produced by defective valves of the heart were cited at the Club (October 1951).[305]

http://www.nasonline.org/publications/biographical-memoirs/memoir-pdfs/wig-gers-carl.pdf

Glossary of terms and notes on the minutes

Acute rheumatism *March 1952* This was usual terminology for an episode of rheumatic fever.[306] See also Rheumatic, also Rheumatic fever.

Angiocardiography *June 1948, May 1949 and generally.* This means taking pictures while the blood passing through the heart contains fluid which will show on x-rays. A history of angiocardiography[307] states that Tom Hills and the cardiologist Dr Maurice Campbell were important in its development, citing their publications.[71;177] Most of these angiocardiograms were performed by injection of contrast medium in peripheral veins or through catheters advanced towards but usually still outside the heart.[307] Ian Hill recorded that The veins of choice are the basilic at the right elbow, the cephalic in the right upper arm or at the right elbow, or the similar veins in the left arm.[51] Angiocardiography was the subject of the meeting in *May 1949* when Dr Campbell gave a review of the first 50 angiocardiograms performed at Guys with Dr Frances Gardner[222] present. Further discussions were had in *December 1949* and *February 1950*. In *July 1951* Reynolds presented the findings of a study of electrocardiography during angiocardiography prompted by three deaths shortly after the procedure. Reynolds study and two earlier studies about deaths and complications were published in the *BHJ* and the *BMJ*.[68;71;72]

Aortic incompetence *December 1954* Back flow or leak of the valve, also called regurgitation.

Aortic stenosis *May 1954, December 1955* Narrowing of the aortic valve. This was the main subject for discussion in the Club on the above two dates.

Aschoff nodes *May 1951 and March 1952* A histological appearance associated with rheumatic fever described in Conybeare 1949 as localised collections of large branching cells with multiple nuclei.[4]

Ballistocardiography *November 1953* A technique for producing a graphical representation of repetitive motions of the human body arising from the sudden ejection of blood into the great vessels with each heartbeat.

Barts *November 1953* St Bartholomews Hospital across the river from Guys. Ian Hill was consultant there by this time.

Blalock operation *February 1953* Appeared in the standard text book Conybeare in 1949.[4] ... Blalock and Taussig have introduced an operation which by an anastomosis between the subclavian and pulmonary artery carries more blood to the lungs for oxygenation and greatly alleviates the symptoms (p.243).

Bleeding *July 1948* Also called venesection. In this context bleeding refers to therapeutic removal of a quantity of blood to reduce the red cell mass. As the body compensates for the lost volume, the red cells are diluted down and the bloods viscosity (their term) is reduced.

Bing test *April 1949* The test involved measuring the patients oxygen from a gas-filled bag and measuring the oxygen content of arterial blood and mixed venous blood and deducing the cardiac output.[55] It relies on the Fick principle. In patients with Fallots Tetralogy Bing derived an estimate of the pulmonary blood flow.[53]

Cardiac catheterisation *June 1948* Here right heart catheterisation is the starting point. This entails passing a fine tube into a peripheral vein and threading it towards the heart, to sample blood to test its oxygen content and to measure pressures. This is technically distinct from angiocardiography when radio-opaque liquids are injected to get contrast pictures showing up the heart and central vessels. The two can be done at the same intervention but there were demarcations in some hospitals. The distinction being made between catheterisation and angiocardiography in the minutes of *June*

1848 might have been because contrast was injected into a peripheral vein avoiding the risks of central catheterision.[51;72;228]

Cerebral thrombosis *July 1948* See also Thrombosis. In his textbook, Conybeare[4] made the distinction between embolism in which the thrombus is carried in the blood stream and thrombosis in which it occurs in situ. The distinction was clearly being made by Dr McArdle at this meeting.

Cirrhosis of the liver *June 1948* Degenerative liver disease. Using Conybeare as a contemporary source the context here is that ... inability of the right ventricle to maintain the circulation efficiently results in typical pathological changes in practically all the organs of the body; such changes are the same whatever the cause of the failure, whether associated with valvular disease or due entirely to myocardial disease. Owing to the condition of general venous stasis, characteristic changes occur in the liver ... the outer zones of the lobule are yellow from fatty degeneration. P.413[4] ... a yellow or tawny appearance from which the name cirrhosis is derived. P345[4]

Coarctation *February 1955* It was the main topic for discussion. Coarctation is narrowing of the aorta, typically at the uppermost part of the descending aorta.

Complete cases *June 1948 and repeatedly later* The Club members correlated post mortem (autopsy, necropsy) examination of the heart with their clinical, catheterisation and/or operative findings and thus they had the complete case. Kazuo Ishiguro uses the words complete/completion/completed for the death of the cloned young people of his novel after their final, fatal organ donation.[308;309]

Congenital morbus cordis *June 1948* This is Latin meaning disease of the heart present at birth. It was custom to use such phrases in no small part because it was intended to not be understood if used in the presence of the patient and family.

Cor pulmonale *February 1951* Where there is severe lung disease, resistance to blood flow may result in higher pulmonary artery pressure and progressive changes to the right ventricle, right atrium and venous engorgement. The term is not indexed by Lewis or Conybeare.

Coronary thrombosis *December 1954* This means a clot in a coronary artery, that is the artery supplying the heart muscle. As a concept it has come in and out of acceptance although the benefit of thrombolysis in clinical trials seemed to settle the matter. The terminology related to coronary heart disease, and its framing as disease, changed during the course of the twentieth century as described in the historical analysis by Christopher Lawrence published in 1992.[310]

Cyanotic *Throughout the Minutes* Cyanosis is the blueness around the lips seen if the arterial blood is not replete with oxygen. In this context, it indicates any form of congenital heart disease where the deoxygenated (blue) blood which should be returned to the lungs for oxygenation, mixes with blood to the rest of the body. The interpretation was made more difficult if lung disease was also present providing a pulmonary factor to the cyanosis. Acyanotic means without cyanosis indicating a simple dichotomy in the contemporary taxonomy of congenital heart disease as seen in Campbells lecture and his chapter in Conybeare.[16;17]

Cyclopropane *December 1953, February 1954* An anaesthetic agent introduced in the 1930s. There was concern that it might be a cause of ventricular fibrillation but Dr Rink thought not if it was properly used.

Cyprus *November 1948* There were several British hospitals in Cyprus. It is not clear what this relationship was but it is evident from this minute that there were patients referred from Cyprus.
http://www.qaranc.co.uk/bmhnicosia.php

Development, embryology, comparative anatomy *January 1949* Campbell arranged for the Club to devote a meeting to the embryological development of the heart with a noted embryologist Willis,[271] and Foxon[216-219] from Guys Biology department.

Dicoumarol *July 1949* An oral anticoagulant.

Digitalis *November 1950* Digitalis is an alkaloid from the foxglove *Digitalis purpurea* used to slow the fast heart rate associated with atrial fibrillation. Conybeare devoted a page to the various preparations: powdered leaves, a tincture or the extract known as digoxin.[4]

Diodone *November 1948* An iodine containing radiocontrast material.

Direct cardiac operations *November 1948 and repeated later* The Brock procedure was on the obstruction itself, that is the pulmonary valve and/or the infundibulum, and so direct as opposed to Blalocks and Potts indirect operation in which blood is redirected from the systemic to the pulmonary circulation downstream of the pulmonary valve.[144]

Douglas bag *March 1952* An inflatable bag with a breathing tube and valve such that expired gas is collected over a period and then analysed. Used in the Bing test.

Dye was used in two senses. It is an informal word for contrast medium used in radiography. A blue dye was used for dye dilution tests to estimate blood flow.

Ductus *December 1948* The ductus arteriosus is part of the foetal circulation allowing a free flow of blood from the pulmonary artery to bypass the uninflated lungs and join the systemic circulation beyond the arteries to the head and upper body. If it fails to close after birth (the usual occurrence) it is called persistent or patent ductus arteriosus abbreviated to PDA. Amongst Club members the ductus used in context, needs no qualifiers. Closed naturally it becomes a fibrous band, an anatomical structure called the ligamentum arteriosum. Of special importance here is that if the ductus remains open blood can pass from the aorta to the pulmonary artery. That additional anomaly can be lifesaving when the normal route is denied by pulmonary atresia or severe stenosis. It was Helen Taussigs observation that lead her to ask Blalock could you make me a ductus? That is what Vivien Thomas achieved in the laboratory.

The Heart Club

Ebstein malformation *March 1949* This does not appear in Conybeare. It was described by Wilhelm Ebstein in 1866 as a very rare case of insufficiency of the tricuspid valve caused by a congenital malformation.

Eisenmenger syndrome *April 1949* When there is a communication between the systemic and the pulmonary circulations at atrial, ventricular level, or through a ductus arteriosus, and there is an excessive flow through the lungs, this may cause the lung vascular resistance to rise (pulmonary vascular disease) and the shunt reverses. The description has been attributed to Woods paper in 1958[311] but it appears in the Club minutes well before that. Elsewhere in the Minutes Eisenmengers complex is written and I am unsure if they use the terms interchangeably. In January 1956 Brock said, in the context of overriding aorta that it was confusing mumbojumbo but quite what and why may have been lost in the process of writing the Minutes.

Electrocardiogram *Generally* The electrical activity of the heart is detected by skin (surface) electrodes. In December 1948 Brock asked that a further attempt should be made to solve the problems of obtaining satisfactory electrocardiograms during operations and here he meant hot wire record on heat sensitive paper strip. This gave way in due course to the ubiquitous screen display familiar to all. A good ECG recording required expertise to acquire. Harken specifically mentions its use in his series of operations to remove bullets and shrapnel from injured servicemen at the US military hospital in Cirencester UK: Throughout these operations electrocardiograms have been taken ...[14] Pictures in Conybeare those are Campbells hand-picked illustrations for textbook publication, had a lot of electrical noise.[4] See for example the illustration related to John Huntss electric shock, administered by Donald Ross, to halt ventricular tachycardia.[99] The ECG was discussed again at length in July 1951.

Fairchild camera *February 1950, March 1951* Cameras made for aerial photography with a high shutter speed to cope with the movement of the plane, and film on a roll rather than individual plates. These features were also useful in taking x-ray pictures of the contrast circulating through the heart and great vessels. Hills had purchased in 1951 a Fairchild roll film camera, previously used by the US Airforce for aerial reconnaissance during the war, that was fitted beneath an ordinary fluorographic table. This produced films of 9.5 x 9.5 at 2 per second, suitable for the young and adolescent heart ... [307] Hills told the Club it was available in March 1951 meeting.

Fallot's Tetralogy *Generally* Described in Conybeare 1949 as a mixture of pulmonary stenosis, a ventricular septal defect, an aorta overriding the septum which allows blood from the right ventricle to reach the aorta, and right ventricular hypertrophy. This combination has been known as Fallots Tetralogy though it might have been called after Peacock, who gave an excellent description of all these points, and who realised its frequency. [4]

Fibrillation *Generally* Commonly as a short form for auricular fibrillation. My contemporary source is Conybeare 1949: Auricular fibrillation, whether paroxysmal or permanent, may be a feature of almost any form of heart disease. Before middle age its incidence is greatest as a sequel of rheumatic carditis, and it is particularly common in patients with mitral stenosis. [4] When fibrillation is used without qualification and particularly in the context of mitral valve disease and other rheumatic heart disease, this is what they are referring to. The word atrial is nowadays used in exactly the same sense. Because auricle was used by the ancients, likening the atrial appendage to an earlobe, the chamber as a whole was referred to by that name in the Minutes. As the terminology of cardiac anatomy began to matter more because operations could be performed, there is a distinction made between the atrium as a whole and it auricular appendage, both on the left and the right. See *ventricular* fibrillation separately.

Fick principle *November 1953* The essence of the Fick principle is that blood flow to an organ can be calculated if the amount of marker substance taken up or released by an organ per unit time can be measured, and the concentration of the marker substance in arterial blood supplying the organ and its concentration in venous blood leaving the organ. In Ficks original method, the organ was the entire human body and the marker substance was oxygen.

Foramen ovale *March 1949* A communication between the right and left atria, normal in the foetal circulation, allowing oxygenated placental blood to cross to the left side. At birth a rise in pressure normally closes the flap like opening. In about 15% of people an opening remains allowing intermittent right to left communication and these people are vulnerable to venous thrombus that would be filtered by the lung, crossing in the heart to emerge in the arterial blood causing a stroke. See also paradoxical embolus.

Gibbon heart lung machine *March 1955* This was used for the first time with success in May 1953 to close an interauricalar septal defect in May 1953.[312] Gibbon had been experimenting in the animals since the 1930s. He had several deaths in patients and, despite one success, he decided not to continue. John Kirklin at the Mayo Clinic took up the challenge and reported some surviving patients in 1955.[313] In 1956, there were 24 surviving patients out of 40 operations.[314]

Gum acacia *July 1948* Alternatives to blood for expanding or replacing the circulating blood volume were in use at the time. Nowadays their merits remain a matter of debate in surgical physiology. The origin of gum acacia is indicated in this MRC note from 1917: Bayliss recently drew attention to the importance of viscosity in solutions used to replace blood lost by haemorrhage. He considered that gum acacia was a suitable substance to add to saline for such purposes, as imparting the requisite viscosity and as being a colloid with a definite osmotic pressure.[315] Brock was particularly interested in surgical physiology and the management of blood volume and peripheral resistance and was still researching and publishing original work while I was a student at Guys.[327]

Hilar dance *February* 1951 The appearance on fluoroscopy of the pulmonary arteries when there is a left to right shunt and very much increased pulmonary blood flow.

Homograft *October 1952* Standard usage then for a graft from the same species – human to human in this instance.

Icterus *July* 1948 Conybeare referred his readers to jaundice for which icterus is a synonym.[4]

Hypothermia. *March 1956* At about 30°c the circulation was stopped by clamping the veins returning to the right atrium so halting the circulation.

Tom Treasure

This allowed up to about five minutes which was long enough to suture an ostium secundum ASD. See the illustration of a patient in a cold bath from the late Ian Hills collection of photographs taken at Guys. Thomas Holmes Sellors at The Middlesex Hospital was an acknowledged master of this technique [316]

Infundibulum *June 1949* By infundibulum, Brock was referring to the conical part of the right ventricle and its outflow to the pulmonary artery. Campbell had proposed that infundibular was used rather than subvalvular for narrowing at this site (December 1948). It was also discussed at the January 1949 with Willis and Foxon.

Johns Hopkins Hospital *Repeatedly* There was an arrangement between Johns Hopkins Hospital in Baltimore and Guys, for exchange of senior members of staff, funded by the Company of Clothworkers.[317] Blalock in 1947, Campbells visit in September 1948, and Brocks visit in 1949 (referred to in the February 1950 Minutes) were a result of the arrangement.

Laparoscopy *June 1948* Direct visual inspection of the abdominal cavity with a narrow illuminated telescope inserted through the skin. It was an application of the thoracoscope used to enable artificial pneumothorax for collapse therapy when adhesions held the lung up. Conybeare advises the help of a surgeon should be invoked for the direct examination of ... adhesions through the thoracoscope, so that he may proceed to divide them with cautery.[4]

Lipoid *November 1948* Related to lipids, including fats and oils.

Membership of the Peacock Club *November 1948* Reading and rereading the Minutes there seems to be some flexibility in who were to be designated as members. After a meeting at the Royal Society of Medicine Brock wrote at Guys there is a group of some 15 people actively engaged in the work[1] and readers of the Minutes will see who they are from the listing of attendees in the early years. In addition residents, clinical fellows and research fellows were *ex officio* members. In December 1950 Mr Barrett asked a question on the subject of nature of the Peacock Club & visitors & Dr Campbell in replying indicated the essentially Guys nature of the club.

Later the names were no longer recorded and any later distinction between members and guests cannot be made from the Minutes.

Mitral *June 1948 and repeatedly* Related to the mitral valve. The non-return valve between the left atrium and ventricle was likened to a mitre, a bishops hat, because of its two leaflets or flaps.

Mitral stenosis *September 1948, September* 1950 The stated concern of the Club was the management of Congenital disease of the Heart but Brock wrote in 1948 When one examines the heart post mortem in patients dying of valvular disease and contemplates the minute size of the orifice through which the whole life blood of the body has to be forced it is impossible not to feel that this simple mechanical obstruction must be capable of relief by surgery. He was not limiting his statement to congenital pulmonary stenosis. Within months of the Club starting Dr Zak presented the cardiac catheterisation report on Doris Diggins (Mitral Stenosis). The Club discussed The policy of refraining from angiocardiography in mitral stenotics within the present limitation of the x-ray generator was explained and Dr Rink commented on the optimum position for anaesthetisation of mitral stenotics undergoing operation. Dr Allanby recorded the circulation times of Doris Diggins and a brief discussion followed on the correlation of these circulatory findings and those shewn in angiocardiography. Doris Diggins had her operation three days later on 16th September and Brock did another mitral dilatation two weeks later. The Guys team did not publish until 1950 by which time there were seven survivors from nine operations (the seventh is added as a footnote, including two at Johns Hopkins.[318] Taken in isolation the statement in September 1950 is misleading: It was decided to include the subject of mitral stenosis and of acquired heart disease generally in the clubs activities. In fact Baker, Brock and Campbell had already published their first paper on successful surgery for mitral stenosis in June 1950.[63] In 1952 they published 100 cases with the highly influential Paul Wood in their company.[118] The Mackenzie Lewis conviction that the trouble in mitral stenosis is the myocardium. It could now be claimed that the source of the trouble in mitral stenosis is mitral stenosis making it an appropriate target for direct surgery on a stenosed heart valve.[45]

Morbus cruleus *June 1949* Heart disease with cyanosis.

Tom Treasure

Oligaemic and pleonaemic *February 1951* Campbell regarded these as his own nomenclature for reduced and increased lung blood flow as interpreted from x-rays. Pleonaemic (excessive blood flow) was used later by Donald Ross.[326] Oligaemic is current usage.

Ostium primum and ostium secundum *March 1956* Embryologically different forms of atrial septal defect.

Pacemaker, stimulator *December 1948* A means of delivering an electrical pulse to the heart to trigger a beat. The request from Brock reminds us that this equipment did not exist as routine equipment and its introduction had to be requested. Pacemakers are now commonplace, routinely available during surgery, and in use in millions of patients as implanted devices.

Paradoxical embolus *July 1948* Defects of the interauricular septum ... may enable an embolus which originated in a peripheral vein to reach a systemic artery with the production of so-called paradoxical embolism. This is quoted directly from Conybeare P.423.[4]

Phonocardiogram *December 1948, December 1955* A means of recording the heart sounds. Conybeare does not mention it. Reinhold who had studied the technique mentioned it in December 1955.[319;320]

Platelet count *July 1948* Particles, smaller than blood cells intimately concerned with coagulation(p.258).[4]

Popliteal emboli *March 1949* The popliteal fossa is the hollow behind the knee and is where the main artery of the thigh branches. At any branching, there is step down in the width of the blood vessel and a thrombus (blood clot) can lodge and obstruct the flow. Reading between the lines the patient probably died of gangrene of both legs.

PM service *June 1948* Post mortem examination of the body after death, autopsy. At the June 1948 meeting Dr Allanby volunteered to establish a travelling P.M. service ... Allanby was 25 at the time and had been qualified for only two years. He was nicknamed the General and this entry suggests why the name stuck.[321] I cannot confirm and I doubt that a travelling autopsy service was actually set up. At the time however, autopsies were much more common and retention of the heart for study would have been unremarkable.

Polycythaemia. *July 1948.* ... a condition in which the number of red corpuscles is increased (p..281).[4] Conybeare used secondary polycythaemia to make the distinction between this finding in cyanotic heart disease and (rubra) vera as a condition in its own right. Under the heading of Fallots Tetralogy (p.423) A few cases survive to adult life ... Their polycythaemia, which increases the appearance of cyanosis, is of course an essential in getting on as well as this.[4]

Potts *November 1953* Potts devised a side to side anastomosis between the descending aorta and the left pulmonary artery as an alternative to Alfred Blalocks subclavian aortic anastomosis and published this operation in 1946.[302]

Precordial beat and feeble pulse *March 1956* Present day expert opinion (Kate Bull[3]) informs me that this is incorrect – the pulses are not weak with an ASD. This illustrates a dilemma in writing history. Their interpretation of physical signs was that with an atrial septal defect a proportion of the oxygenated blood from the lungs takes the path of least resistance into the right atrium and the thin walled right ventricle and is pumped back around the lungs. The flow through the right ventricle is typically about three times that pumped out to the body, hence the forcible beat felt at the front of the chest – the precordium. Dr Campbell and his colleagues perceived that there was a relatively weak arterial pulse. In present day medicine these perceptions can be readily confirmed or refuted on investigation and many physical signs described in earlier days have been found to be unreliable or simply wrong.

Procaine *Repeatedly* Used intravenously or directly onto the heart to reduce the tendency to ventricular arrhythmias.[322]

Pulmonary *Regularly* Anything pertaining to the lungs or the course of blood to and from them.

Tom Treasure

Pulmonary stenosis *Regularly* The pulmonary valve is at the outflow of the right ventricle into the pulmonary artery. ... the stenosis is sometimes valvular and sometimes rather low and infundibular, and these cannot easily be distinguished ... (p.423).[5]

Punch-card system. *April 1948.* Before there were any usable computers for clinical teams this was a widely used means of keeping and extracting data. The patients individual record card had multiple numbered or labelled holes around the margin and for example, by punching out the hole F (but not M) to the cards edge, a rod passed through F would retain all male patients allowing only female patients card to fall out. Similarly decade of age and particular features of the disease could be selected. This was the method used by clinicians to collate data up to the 1970s.[323]

Quinidine *November 1950* ... may be used to abolish atrial fibrillation.[4]

Sanborn *October 1951* Electronic company, later Hewlett-Packard.

Rheumatic fever *March 1952* Dr Baker presented on acute rheumatism in patients with mitral stenosis. Dr Bywaters said all his post mortem studies on acute rheumatic fever in children had shown Aschoff nodes in the heart, but the left auricular appendix had not been examined. He understood by rheumatic activity joint pains and tachycardia. March 1952 The immediate and dramatic effects of cortisone on their painful inflamed joints were confirmed but the important question was did cortisone protect the heart from rheumatic heart disease? The answer five years later was that it did not.[*] Rheumatic fever was a familiar diagnosis at the time and one which has an interesting history in terms of framing disease.[324]

Spirometer *April 1949* A machine to measure volumes of air breathed, against a time base.

Stenosis *Regularly* Narrowing of a valve, blood vessel or any channel.

---

* From the entry on Bywaters in Munks roll http://munksroll.rcplondon.ac.uk/Biography/Details/5148

The Heart Club

Surgical Thoracic Unit *June 1948* Guys was a general hospital and Brock had been appointed as a surgeon to the hospital. The process of specialisation is a big subject in the history of medicine but at the beginning of the time window of the Club in 1948 the clinicians were seeking to mark out and ring fence their facilities as can be seen in the Medical Committee minutes of the time. The qualifying term general surgeon only became necessary after subdivision into specialties. Up to this time Mr Brock had shared ward beds and junior staff with another surgeon and this process of marking out the territory and having his own team was an important step.

St Thomas's Hospital *October 1951, February 1953* I use this punctuation which is not the one preferred by that hospital[325] where that is how it is written in the Minutes.

Sympathectomy and ganglionectomy *November 1953* Interrupting the sympathetic nerve supply to arteries prevents the blood vessels constricting and allows less restricted blood flow.

Transposition *Regularly* A congenital malformation in which the arteries connected to the right and left ventricles are reversed.

Thrombosis *July 1948* Formation of blood clots within the blood vessels is the basis of a wide number of illnesses (coronary thrombosis, deep vein thrombosis). It was discussed by Drs McArdle and Waterfield.

Warden's House *Regularly* Guys was probably unusual in having the post of Warden. Charles Baker held the post for many years. The Club often met there or repaired to the Wardens house, also referred to as Dr Bakers house, after meeting at some place less convivial.

Valvulotomy, valvotomy *Regularly until October 1951* In previous papers we have followed common usage in writing of pulmonary or mitral valvulotomy, but it is a valve and not a valvule that is divided, and we think the term valvotomy is more correct, even though it is still a hybrid formation.[118]

Vegetations *November 1948* These are soft, fragile aggregations of the materials that form blood clots (fibrins and platelets), attached to the heart valves and the lining of the heart. They have a surface texture a bit like a cauli-flower but are usually measured in millimetres. Nowadays they can be seen on an echocardiogram wafting precariously in the blood stream. At the time of the Club, vegetations could only be seen at autopsy. In the context of structural heart disease, they are a hallmark of infection within the heart called endocarditis.

Venesection *September 1948* Removal of a volume of blood from a vein as a treatment. Here they refer to a pint or roughly 10% of the blood volume.

Ventricular fibrillation *February 1954* Uncoordinated and ineffective activity of the heart muscle. Mr Milstein spoke about the subject in February 1954 and wrote on the subject in Guys Hospital Reports.[98]

Ventricular septal defect (VSD) *Regularly but the subject of the meeting in January 1956* An opening in the muscle separating the left and right ventri-cles. It is a component of Fallots Tetralogy.

Abbreviations

ACTH	adrenocorticotrophic hormone
AMC	Alan Mason Chesney
AP	anteroposterior
ASD	atrial septal defect
AV (valve)	atrioventricular
AV (fistula)	arteriovenous
BP	blood pressure
ChM	Master of Surgery
CO_2	carbon dioxide
DA	Diploma of Anaesthesia
DCH	Diploma in Child Health
DMRE	Diploma in Medical Radiology and Electrology
ECG	electrocardiogram which is a graph of voltage against time
EPBF	effective pulmonary blood flow
ESR	erythrocyte sedimentation rate
FFA RCS	Fellow of the Faculty of Anaesthetists of the Royal College of Surgeons
FRCP	Fellow of the Royal College of Physicians
FRCS	Fellow of the Royal College of Surgeons
FRS	Fellow of the Royal Society
GUCH	grown up congenital heart disease
Hb	haemoglobin
Hct	haematocrit
LMSSA	Licentiate in Medicine and Surgery of the Society of Apothecaries
MCHC	mean corpuscular haemoglobin content
MCV	mean corpuscular volume
MGH	Massachusetts General Hospital

ml	millilitre
mmHg	millimetres of mercury as a measure of blood pressure
MRC	Medical Research Council
MRCP	Member of the Royal College of Physicians
MS (in cardiac context)	mitral stenosis
MS (in Biographies)	Master of Surgery
PA (films/x-rays)	postero-anterior
PAP	pulmonary artery pressure
PDA	patent/persistent ductus arteriosus
PFO	patent foramen ovale
pH	measure of acidity
PM	post mortem that is after death
PR (interval)	time between atrial and ventricular activity on the ECG
PVS	pulmonary valve stenosis
QRS	the deflections in the electrocardiogram due to ventricular contraction
QT	deflections in the electrocardiogram due to all ventricular voltage changes
R (wave)	part of the QRS complex in the electrocardiogram
RAD	right axis deviation of the ECG
RAF	Royal Air Force
RAMC	Royal Army Medical Corps
RBC	red blood cell
RPA	right pulmonary artery
RPGMS	Royal Post Graduate Medical School
RV	right ventricle/ventricular
RVP	right ventricular predominance
SD	standard deviation (statistical)
S-T (depression)	the portion of the electrocardiogram between the S and the T waves
T (wave)	the voltage changes associated with ventricular repolarisation
USA	United States of America
V (wave)	a venous pulse wave attributed to the Ventricular contraction

V1	in cardiac context V1-V6 are the chest leads of the ECG
VSD	ventricular septal defect
WW1	1914-1918 war
WW2	1939-1945 war

Reference List

(1) Brock R. Discussion on the surgery of the heart and great vessels. *Proc R Soc Med* 1951; 44(12):995-1003.

(2) Peacock T. On malformations, &c., of the human heart: with original cases. London: John Churchill; 1858.

(3) Bull K. Open Hearts. Stories of the Surgery that Changes Childrens Lives. London: Elliott & Thompson; 2016.

(4) Conybeare J, by Various Authors. Textbook of Medicine. 1st ed. Edinburgh: E&S Livingstone; 1949.

(5) Campbell M, Conybeare J. Congenital Heart Disease. Textbook of Medicine. 9th ed. Edinburgh: E&S Livingstone Ltd; 1949.

(6) Hurt R. The History of Cardiothoracic Surgery from Early Times. 1st ed. Carnforth, Lancashire, UK: Parthenon Publishing Group; 1996.

(7) Editor. Passim: Disinterrment of Thomas Guy from his tomb of concrete. *Guy's Hospital Gazette* 2045; 59(1482 12th May 1945):210-211.

(8) Bishop P. Guys and the German War. *Guy's Hospital Gazette* 1945; 59(1487):172-179.

(9) Brock R. Fractured ribs and other chest injuries. *Guy's Hospital Gazette* 1945; 59(1488 4th August 1945):184-189.

(10) Campbell M. Orpington 1939-1945. *Guy's Hospital Gazette* 1946; 60:29.

(11) Johnston T. Guys and the National Health Service bill. *Guy's Hospital Gazette* 2017; 60(1506 13th April 1946):97-98.

(12) Boland E. Ex-servicemen as House Officers at Guys. *Guy's Hospital Gazette* 1946; 60:159.

(13) Wertenbaker L. To mend the heart. New York: The Viking Press; 1980.

(14) Harken DE. Foreign bodies in, and in relation to, the thoracic blood vessels and the heart. *Surg Gynecol Obstet* 1946; 83:117-125.

(15) Editor. Passim: Alfred Blalock welcomed to Guys. *Guy's Hospital Gazette* 1947; 61(1543 13th September 1947):251-252.

(16) Campbell M, Conybeare J. Congenital Heart Disease. Textbook of Medicine. 8th ed. Edinburgh: E&S Livingstone Ltd; 1946.

(17) Campbell M. Congenital Heart Disease. *Guy's Hospital Gazette* 1946; 50:150-156.

(18) Blalock A, Taussig H. The surgical treatment of malformations of the heart in which there is pulmonary stenosis or pulmonary atresia. *JAMA* 1945; 128:189-202.

(19) Campbell M. The Blalock-Taussig operation for morbus coeruleus. *Guy's Hospital Reports* 1948; 97:1-47.

(20) Taussig H, Blalock A, Brown J, Crafoord C, Gilchrist A, Tubbs O et al. Surgery of congenital heart diseases. *Lancet* 1947; 2(6473):434-435.

(21) Taussig H, Blalock A, Crafoord C, Gilcrist R, Campbell M. Surgery of congenital heart disease. *BMJ* 1947; 2(4524):462-463.

(22) Tubbs O. The effect of ligation on infection of the persistent patent ductus arteriosus. *Br J Surg* 1944; 32:1-12.

(23) Crafoord C, Campbell M. Patent ductus arteriosus and coarctation. *Br Med J* 1947; 2(4524):462.

(24) Taussig H, Blalock A, Brown J, Crafoord C, Gilcrist R, Sellors H et al. The surgery of congenital heart disease. *Br Heart J* 1948; 10(2):65-79.

(25) Atkins H. Department of Surgery. *Guy's Hospital Gazette* 1947; 61:23.

(26) Blalock A, Bahnson H. Operations performed and vascular anomalies encountered in the treatment of congenital pulmonic stenosis. *Ann R Coll Surg Engl* 1948; 3(2):57-76.

(27) Campbell M, Deuchar D, Brock R. Results of pulmonary valvotomy and infundibular resection in 100 cases of Fallots tetralogy. *Br Med J* 1954; 2(4880):111-122.

(28) Campbell M, Deuchar D. Results of the Blalock-Taussig operation in 200 cases of morbus caeruleus. *Br Med J* 1953; 1(4806):349-358.

(29) Sellors TH. Surgery of pulmonary stenosis; a case in which the pulmonary valve was successfully divided. *Lancet* 1948; 1(6513):988.

(30) Brock R. Pulmonary valvulotomy for the relief of congenital pulmonary stenosis; report of three cases. *Br Med J* 1948; 1(4562):1121-1126.

(31) Hollman A, Treasure T. Pulmonary valvotomy--50 years ago. *Lancet* 1998; 352(9145):1956.

(32) Samways DW. Mitral stenosis: a statistical inquiry. *Br Med J* 1898; 1(1936):364-365.

(33) Samways DW. Cardiac peristalsis: its nature and effects. *The Lancet* 1898; i:927.

(34) Brunton L. Preliminary note on the possibility of treating mitral stenosis by surgical methods. *Lancet* 1902; i(8th February 1902):352.

(35) Lancet. Surgical operation for mitral stenosis. *Lancet* 1902; i(15th February 1902):461-462.

(36) Souttar HS. The surgical treatment of mitral stenosis. *BMJ* 1925; ii:603-607.

(37) Ellis RH. Henry Souttar and surgery of the mitral valve. Part I: the surgeon and his patient. *J Med Biogr* 1997; 5(1):8-13.

(38) Ellis RH. Henry Souttar and surgery of the mitral valve. Part II: the operation and its aftermath. *J Med Biogr* 1997; 5(2):63-69.

(39) Cutler EC, Beck CS. Present status of surgical procedures in chronic valvular disease of the heart; final report of all surgical cases. *Arch Surg* 1929; 18:403-416.

(40) Pratt J. Recollections and letters of Sir James Mackenzie. *New England J Med* 1941; 224:1-10.

(41) Mackenzie J. A new outlook in cardiology. *Br Med J* 1924; i(3288):1-5.

(42) Mackenzie J. A new outlook in cardiology. *Br Med J* 1924; i(3289):57-61.

(43) Mackenzie J. A new outlook in cardiology. *Br Med J* 1924; i(3290):104-109.

(44) Cutler E, Levine S. Cardiotomy and valvulotomy for mitral stenosis. Experimental observations and clinical notes concerning an operative case with recovery. *Boston Medical and Surgical Journal* 1923; 188:1023.

(45) McMichael J. A transition in cardiology: the Mackenzie Lewis era. The Harveian Oration of 1975. 1976. London, Royal College of Physicians.

(46) Silverman ME. Maurice Campbell: first editor of Heart. *Heart* 2003; 89(12):1379-1381.

(47) Lewis T. Diseases of the Heart. 3rd ed. London: MacMillan and Co.; 1943.

(48) Bailey C. The surgical treatment of mitral stenosis (mitral commissurotomy). *Dis Chest* 1949; 15(4):377-397.

(49) Harken D, Ellis L. The surgical treatment of mitral stenosis; valvuloplasty. *N Engl J Med* 1948; 239(22):801-809.

(50) Wass S. The Residents Play: a review. *Guy's Hospital Gazette* 1948; 62:159-160.

(51) Hill I. A method of angiocardiography. *Br J Surg* 1953; 40(163):444-446.

(52) Bing R, Vandam L, Gray F. Physiological studies in congenital heart disease. *Bull Johns Hopkins Hosp* 1947; 80(2):107-120.

(53) Bing R, Vandam L, Gray F. Physiological studies in congenital heart disease; results of preoperative studies in patients with tetralogy of Fallot. *Bull Johns Hopkins Hosp* 1947; 80(2):121-141.

(54) Bing R, Vandam L, Gray F. Physiological studies in congenital heart disease: results obtained in five cases of Eisenmengers complex. *Bull Johns Hopkins Hosp* 1947; 80(6):323-347.

(55) Bing R, Vandam L, Gray F. Physiological studies in congenital heart disease. *Bull Johns Hopkins Hosp* 1947; 81(1):74-76.

(56) Bloomfield RA, Lauson HD, Cournand A, Breed ES, Richards DW. Recording of right heart pressures in normal subjects and patients with chronic pulmonary disease and various types of cardio-circulatory disease. *J Clin Invest* 1946; 25(4):639-664.

(57) Knipping H, Moncrieff A. The ventilation equivalent for oxygen. *Quarterly Journal of Medicine* 1932; 1(1):17-30.

(58) Knipping HW. [The sick heart in physical work and athletic exertion, with comments on their therapeutic use]. Munch Med Wochenschr 1950; 92(29-30):1210-1217.

(59) Brock R, Campbell M. Infundibular resection or dilatation for infundibular stenosis. *Br Heart J* 1950; 12(4):403-424.

(60) Brinton W. Haematological changes in cases of congenital cyanotic heart disease which have been submitted to operations designed to improve the circulation to the lungs: Part I. *Guys Hosp Rep* 1951; 100(1-2):148-183.

(61) Brinton W. Haematological changes in cases of congenital cyanotic heart disease which have been submitted to operations designed to improved the circulation to the lungs: Part II. *Guys Hosp Rep* 1951; 100(3):185-209.

(62) Brinton W. Haematological changes in cases of congenital cyanotic heart disease which have been submitted to operations designed to improve the circulation to the lungs. Part III. Post-operative estimations and discussion of results. *Guys Hosp Rep* 1951; 100(4):283-303.

(63) Baker C, Brock R, Campbell M. Valvulotomy for mitral stenosis. Report of six successful cases. *BMJ* 1950; i:1283-1293.

(64) Bailey C, Glover J, ONeill T, Redondo Ramirez H. Experiences with the experimental surgical relief of aortic stenosis; a preliminary report. *J Thorac Surg* 1950; 20(4):516-541.

(65) ONeill T, Glover R, Bailey C. Commissurotomy for mitral stenosis. *J Int Coll Surg* 1950; 13(4):355-360.

(66) Bailey C, Glover R, ONeill T. The surgery of mitral stenosis. *J Thorac Surg* 1950; 19(1):16-49, illust.

(67) Campbell M. Visible pulsation in relation to blood flow and pressure in the pulmonary artery. *Br Heart J* 1951; 13(4):438-456.

(68) Reynolds G. The electrocardiogram during angiocardiography. *Br Heart J* 1953; 15(1):74-82.

(69) Trounce J. The electrocardiogram in mitral stenosis. *Br Heart J* 1952; 14(2):185-192.

(70) McMillan I, Daley R, Matthews M. The movement of aortic and pulmonary valves studied post mortem by colour cinematography. *Br Heart J* 1952; 14(1):42-46.

(71) Campbell M, Hills T. Angiocardiography in cyanotic congenital heart disease. *Br Heart J* 1950; 12(1):65-95, illust.

(72) Carnegie D. Angiocardiography in congenital heart disease; anaesthesia and technique. *Br Med J* 1951; 1(4717):1230-1233.

(73) Enticknap J. Biopsy of the left auricle in mitral stenosis. *Br Heart J* 1953; 15(1):37-46.

(74) Enticknap J. Lung biopsy in mitral stenosis. *J Clin Pathol* 1953; 6(1):84-88.

(75) Enticknap J, Milstein B, Baker C. Lingular biopsy in mitral stenosis. *Thorax* 1954; 9(1):58-62.

(76) Deuchar D, Zak G. Cardiac catheterization in congenital heart disease. Part I. *Guys Hosp Rep* 1952; 101(1):1-22.

(77) Deuchar D. Cardiac catheterisation in congenital heart disease. Part II Direct domonstration of a singleventricle. *Guy's Hospital Reports* 1952; 101:23-31.

(78) Deuchar D, Knebel R. The pulmonary and systemic circulations in congenital heart disease. *Br Heart J* 1952; 14(2):225-249.

(79) Brunnen P. The preparation and preservation of arterial homografts. *Guys Hosp Rep* 1953; 102(3):194-203.

(80) McMillan I. Aortic stenosis; a post-mortem cinephotographic study of valve action. *Br Heart J* 1955; 17(1):56-62.

(81) Ross D. Hypothermia Part I. A technique of blood stream cooling. *Guys Hosp Rep* 1954; 103(2):97-115.

(82) Ross D. Hypothermia Part II. Physiological observations during hypothermia. *Guys Hosp Rep* 1954; 103(2):116-138.

(83) Ross D. Venous cooling: a new method of cooling the blood-stream. *Lancet* 1954; 266(6822):1108-1109.

(84) Juvenelle A. Observations on hypothermia. *Proc R Soc Med* 1954; 47(6):410-415.

(85) Shephard R. The effect of carbon dioxide on the pulmonary circulation in congenital heart disease. *Br Heart J* 1954; 16(4):451-456.

(86) Shephard R. Pulmonary arterial pressure in acyanotic congenital heart disease. *Br Heart J* 1954; 16(4):361-374.

(87) Shephard R. Haemodynamic instability in Fallots tetralogy. *Guys Hosp Rep* 1954; 103(3):269-273.

(88) Shephard R. Pneumotachographic measurement of breathing capacity. *Thorax* 1955; 10(3):258-268.

(89) Shephard R. The immediate metabolic effects of breathing carbon dioxide mixtures. *J Physiol* 1955; 129(2):393-407.

(90) Shephard R. The carbon dioxide balance-sheets of the body: their determination in normal subjects and in cases of congenital heart disease. *J Physiol* 1955; 129(1):142-158.

(91) Shephard R. The atrial pressure tracing in congenital heart disease. *Br Heart J* 1955; 17(2):225-228.

(92) Shephard R. The resting hyperventilation of congenital heart disease. *Br Heart J* 1955; 17(2):153-162.

(93) Shephard R. A critical examination of the Douglas bag technique. *J Physiol* 1955; 127(3):515-524.

(94) Shephard R. Respiratory responses to the inhalation of oxygen at atmospheric pressure in normal subjects and in cases of congenital heart disease. *J Physiol* 1955; 127(3):498-514.

(95) Shephard R. Pulmonary arterial pressures in persistent ductus arteriosus with particular reference to older patients. *Guys Hosp Rep* 1955; 104(1):46-50.

(96) Shephard R. Redistribution of systemic blood flow in pulmonary stenosis. *Br Heart J* 1955; 17(1):98-104.

(97) Shephard R, Venner A. The pattern of respiration in rheumatic heart disease. *Br Heart J* 1956; 18(2):241-247.

(98) Milstein B, Brock R. Ventricular fibrillation during cardiac surgery. *Guys Hosp Rep* 1954; 103(3):213-259.

(99) McDonald L, Resnekov L, Ross D. Resistant ventricular tachycardia a year after surgical correction of Fallots tetralogy, treated by external electrical countershock. *Lancet* 1963; 2(7310):708-709.

(100) Venner A, Holling H. Comparison of operation and clinical findings in mitral stenosis and incompetence. *Br Heart J* 1953; 15(2):205-213.

(101) Holling H, Venner A. Disability and circulatory changes in mitral stenosis. *Br Heart J* 1956; 18(1):103-122.

(102) Brock R. Surgical treatment of aortic stenosis. *Br Med J* 1957; 1(5026):1019-1028.

(103) Baker C, Brock R, Campbell M. Mitral valvotomy: a follow-up of 45 patients for three years and over. *Br Med J* 1955; 2(4946):983-991.

(104) Baylis J, Campbell M. The course and prognosis of coarctation of the aorta. *Br Heart J* 1956; 18(4):475-495.

(105) Brock R, Milstein B, Ross DN. Percutaneous left ventricular puncture in the assessment of aortic stenosis. *Thorax* 1956; 11(3):163-171.

(106) Brotmacher L, Campbell M. The natural history of ventricular septal defect. *Br Heart J* 1958; 20(1):97-116.

(107) Campbell M. Natural history of ventricular septal defect. *Br Heart J* 1971; 33(2):246-257.

(108) Campbell M, Neill C, Suzman S. The prognosis of atrial septal defect. *Br Med J* 1957; 1(5032):1375-1383.

(109) Reinhold J, Rudhe U. Relation of the first and second heart sounds to events in the cardiac cycle. *Br Heart J* 1957; 19(4):473-485.

(110) Abrahams D. The Q-T interval in acute rheumatic carditis. *Br Heart J* 1949; 11(4):342-349.

(111) Allanby K. Circulation times in congenital heart disease. *Br Heart J* 1949; 11(2):165-169.

(112) Allanby K, Campbell M. Congenital pulmonary stenosis with closed ventricular septal defect. *Guy's Hospital Reports* 1949; 98:18-53.

(113) Allanby K, Brinton W, Campbell M, Gardner F. Pulmonary atresia and the collateral circulation to the lungs. *Guys Hosp Rep* 1950; 99(2-3):110-152.

The Heart Club

(114) Baker C, Brock R. Morbus coeruleus; a study of 50 cases after the Blalock-Taussig operation. *Br Heart J* 1949; 11(2):170-198.

(115) Baker C, Brock R, Campbell M, Suzman S, Zak G. Morbus coeruleus; a study of 50 cases after the Blalock-Taussig operation. *Br Heart J* 1949; 11(2):170-198.

(116) Baker C, Trounce J. Arteriovenous aneurysm of the lung. *Br Heart J* 1949; 11(2):109-118.

(117) Baker C, Brinton W, Channell G. Ebsteins disease. *Guys Hosp Rep* 1950; 99(4):247-275.

(118) Baker C, Brock R, Campbell M, Wood P. Valvotomy for mitral stenosis. A further report, on 100 cases. *BMJ* 1952; i:1043-1055.

(119) Bahnson H, Baker C. Study of prosthetic materials used inside the heart. *Surg Forum* 1953; 4:78-83.

(120) Baker C, Campbell M. The results of valvotomy for aortic stenosis. *Lancet* 1956; 270(6909):171-175.

(121) Baker C, Robinson B, Trounce J. Ventricular tachycardia and fibrillation following quinidine. *Guys Hosp Rep* 1956; 105(4):433-440.

(122) Barrett N, Daley R. A method of increasing the lung blood supply in cyanotic congenital heart disease. *Br Med J* 1949; 1(4607):699-702.

(123) Baylis J, Campbell M. An unusual cause for a continuous murmur. *Guys Hosp Rep* 1952; 101(3):174-185.

(124) Baylis J, Campbell M, Gilmore H, Hudson R. Two cases of ventricular septal defect with over-riding aorta. *Guys Hosp Rep* 1955; 104(2):114-129.

(125) Brinton W. Primary pulmonary hypertension. *Br Heart J* 1950; 12(3):305-311.

(126) Brinton W. Haematological changes in cases of congenital cyanotic heart disease which have been submitted to operations designed to improve the circulation to the lungs. *Guys Hosp Rep* 1951; 100(1-2):148-183.

(127) Brinton W. Haematological changes in cases of congenital cyanotic heart disease which have been submitted to operations designed to improved the circulation to the lungs--Part II. *Guys Hosp Rep* 1951; 100(3):185-209.

(128) Brinton W. Haematological changes in cases of congenital cyanotic heart disease which have been submitted to operations designed to

improve the circulation to the lungs; III. Post-operative estimations and discussion of results. *Guys Hosp Rep* 1951; 100(4):283-303.

(129) Brock R. The surgery of the heart. *Practitioner* 1949; 162(968):122-126.

(130) Brock R. Congenital cyanotic heart disease. *Ir J Med Sci* 1949;(283):305-314.

(131) Brock R. The surgery of pulmonary stenosis. *Br Med J* 1949; 2(4624):399-406.

(132) Brock R. The surgery of the heart. *Practitioner* 1949; 162(968):122-126.

(133) Brock R. The arterial route to the aortic and pulmonary valves. The mitral route to the aortic valves. *Guys Hosp Rep* 1950; 99(4):236-246.

(134) Brock R. [Surgery of the heart]. Minerva Med 1950; 41(36):103-108.

(135) Brock R. [Surgery in stenosis of the pulmonary artery]. Dia Med 1950; 22(42):1663-1675.

(136) Brock R, Campbell M. Valvulotomy for pulmonary valvular stenosis. *Br Heart J* 1950; 12(4):377-402.

(137) Brock R, Campbell M. Valvulotomy for pulmonary valvular stenosis. *Br Heart J* 1950; 12(4):377-402.

(138) Brock R. Cardiac surgery. *Ann R Coll Surg Engl* 1951; 9(1):1-12.

(139) Crafoord C, Brock R, Campbell M. Surgery of the Heart and Great Vessels. *BMJ* 1951; i:946-947.

(140) Brock R, Price Thomas C, Tubbs O, Holmes Sellors T. Cardiac Surgery. *BMJ* 1951; ii:297.

(141) Brock R, Graham J. Resection of combined aneurysm and coarctation of the aorta with insertion of a homograft. *Guys Hosp Rep* 1952; 101(3):207-215.

(142) Brock R. Valvotomy in pregnancy. *Proc R Soc Med* 1952; 45(8):538-540.

(143) Brock R. The surgical and pathological anatomy of the mitral valve. *Br Heart J* 1952; 14(4):489-513.

(144) Brock R. Direct cardiac surgery in the treatment of congenital pulmonary stenosis. *Ann Surg* 1952; 136(1):63-72.

(145) Brock R. Congenital pulmonary stenosis. *Am J Med* 1952; 12(6):706-719.

(146) Brock R, Rob C, Forty F. Discussion on reconstructive arterial surgery. *Proc R Soc Med* 1953; 46(2):115-130.

The Heart Club

(147) Brock R. Aortic homografting; a report of six successful cases. *Guys Hosp Rep* 1953; 102(3):204-228.

(148) Brock R. Mechanical principles in the surgery of aortic and mitral incompetence. *Br Heart J* 1954; 16(3):317-323.

(149) Brock R, Whytehead L. Radical pneumonectomy for bronchial carcinoma. *Br J Surg* 1955; 43(177):8-24.

(150) Brock R. Direct operations in the treatment of pulmonary stenosis. *Br Med Bull* 1955; 11(3):189-192.

(151) Brock R. Control mechanisms in the outflow tract of the right ventricle in health and disease. *Guys Hosp Rep* 1955; 104(4):356-379.

(152) Brock R, Ross D. Hypothermia. III. The clinical application of hypothermic techniques. *Guys Hosp Rep* 1955; 104(2):99-113.

(153) Brock R, Fleming P. Aortic subvalvar stenosis. *Guy's Hospital Reports* 1956; 105(4):391-408.

(154) Brock R. The technique of mitral valvotomy. *Ann R Coll Surg Engl* 1956; 19(1):1-22.

(155) Brock R. Hypothermia and open cardiotomy. *Proc R Soc Med* 1956; 49(6):347-352.

(156) Brock R, Fleming P. Aortic subvalvar stenosis; a report of 5 cases diagnosed during life. *Guys Hosp Rep* 1956; 105(4):391-408.

(157) Brock R. The surgical approach to the left atrium: removal of an atrial myxoma. *Guys Hosp Rep* 1956; 105(4):382-390.

(158) Brotmacher L, Deuchar D. The systemic blood flow in congenital heart disease, with an examination of the validity of the cardiac index. *Clin Sci* 1956; 15(3):441-456.

(159) Brotmacher L, Fleming P. Cardiac output and vascular pressures in 10 normal children and adolescents. *Guys Hosp Rep* 1957; 106(4):268-272.

(160) Brotmacher L, Fleming P. The diagnosis by cardiac catheterization of superior mediastinal anomalous pulmonary veins. *Guys Hosp Rep* 1957; 106(4):264-267.

(161) Brotmacher L. Haemodynamic effects of squatting during recovery from exertion. *Br Heart J* 1957; 19(4):567-573.

(162) Brotmacher L. Haemodynamic effects of squatting during repose. *Br Heart J* 1957; 19(4):559-566.

(163) Brotmacher L. Medical practice among the Somalis. *Bull Hist Med* 1955; 29(3):197-229.

(164) Brunnen P. Aortic aneurysms. *J R Coll Surg Edinb* 1957; 3(1):41-45.

(165) Bywaters E. The relation between heart and joint disease including rheumatoid heart disease and chronic post rheumatic arthritis (Type Jaccoud). *Br Heart J* 1950; 12(2):101-131.

(166) Bywaters E. The general management of rheumatic fever. *Proc R Soc Med* 1950; 43(3):199-206.

(167) Bywaters E. The bearing of recent advances on the etiology and treatment of rheumatic fever. *Practitioner* 1951; 166(991):14-21.

(168) Bywaters E. Aetiological factors in rheumatic heart disease. *Br Med Bull* 1952; 8(4):343-348.

(169) Campbell M. Natural history of persistent ductus arteriosus. *Br Heart J* 1968; 30(1):4-13.

(170) Campbell M. The natural history of congenital aortic stenosis. *Br Heart J* 1968; 30(4):514-526.

(171) Campbell M. Natural history of congenital pulmonary stenosis. *Br Heart J* 1969; 31(3):394.

(172) Campbell M. Natural history of coarctation of the aorta. *Br Heart J* 1970; 32(5):633-640.

(173) Campbell M. Natural history of atrial septal defect. *Br Heart J* 1970; 32(6):820-826.

(174) Campbell M. Natural history of cyanotic malformations and comparison of all common cardiac malformations. *Br Heart J* 1972; 34(1):3-8.

(175) Campbell M, Suzman S. Coarctation of the aorta. *Br Heart J* 1947; 9(3):185-212.

(176) Campbell M. Surgery of congenital heart disease. *Br Med J* 1948; 2(4579):669-671.

(177) Campbell M, Hills T, Zak GA. Angiocardiography in congenital heart disease. *Br Heart J* 1949; 11(1):97.

(178) Blalock A, Kieffer R, Valvulotomy for the relief of congenital valvular pulmonic stenosis with intact ventricular septum; report of 19 operations by the Brock method. *Trans Meet Am Surg Assoc Am Surg Assoc* 1950;68:176-196.

(179) Campbell M, Hudson R. Patent ductus arteriosus with reversed shunt due to pulmonary hypertension. *Guys Hosp Rep* 1951; 100(1-2):26-44.

(180) Campbell M, Suzman S. Transposition of the aorta and pulmonary artery. *Circulation* 1951; 4(3):329-342.

The Heart Club

(181) Campbell M, Hudson R. The disappearance of the continuous murmur of patent ductus arteriosus. *Guys Hosp Rep* 1952; 101(1):32-44.

(182) Campbell M, Reynolds G, Trounce J. Six cases of single ventricle with pulmonary stenosis. *Guys Hosp Rep* 1953; 102(2):99-139.

(183) Campbell M, Cardell B. A case of Eisenmengers complex with coarctation of the aorta. *Guys Hosp Rep* 1953; 102(4):327-336.

(184) Campbell M, Jackson J. An unusual case of cor biloculare with bilateral superior venae cavae. *Guys Hosp Rep* 1953; 102(4):337-349.

(185) Brinton W, Campbell M. Necropsies in some congenital diseases of the heart, mainly Fallots tetralogy. *Br Heart J* 1953; 15(3):335-349.

(186) Campbell M, Brock R. The results of valvotomy for simple pulmonary stenosis. *Br Heart J* 1955; 17(2):229-246.

(187) Campbell M. Acyanotic congenital heart disease. *Guy's Hospital Gazette* 1956; 70:246-256.

(188) Campbell M, MacCarthy D. Morbus coeruleus with inversion of the abdominal viscera in two cousins. *Guys Hosp Rep* 1957; 106(1):18-28.

(189) Campbell M, Hudson R. A case of Taussig-Bing transposition with survival for 34 years. *Guys Hosp Rep* 1958; 107(1):14-22.

(190) Campbell M, Missen G. Survival in good health until 65 years with pulmonary valvar stenosis. *Guys Hosp Rep* 1959; 108:390-402.

(191) Braithwaite F, Channell G, Moore.F, Whillis J. The applied anatomy of the lumbrical and interosseus muscles of the hand. *Guys Hosp Rep* 1948; 97:185-195.

(192) Channell G, Whillis J. The effect of ulnar nerve block at the level of the pisiform bone on movements of the ring finger. *J Anat* 1949; 83(Pt 1):71.

(193) Whillis J, Channell G. The action of the lumbrical and interosseous muscles in some of the movements of the digits. *J Anat* 1949; 83(Pt 1):60.

(194) Chesterman J, Whitaker W. Mitral and tricuspid valvotomy for mitral and tricuspid stenosis. *Am Heart J* 1954; 48(4):631-636.

(195) Chesterman J, Whitaker W. Surgical treatment of acquired tricuspid stenosis. *Thorax* 1955; 10(4):321-326.

(196) Chesterman J. A new valvulotome. *Lancet* 1955; 269(6883):232.

(197) Chesterman J, Das J. Aneurysms of the patent ductus arteriosus. *Thorax* 1956; 11(4):295-302.

(198) Cleland W, Melrose D. The artificial heart-lung and its practical application to cardiac surgery. *Br Med Bull* 1955; 11(3):236-239.

(199) Cooley DA, DeBakey ME. Surgical treatment of mitral and aortic stenosis: results of one hundred fifteen valvotomies. *J Am Med Assoc* 1954; 155(3):235-239.

(200) Cosh J. Patent ductus arteriosus; a follow-up study of 73 cases. *Br Heart J* 1957; 19(1):13-22.

(201) Bing R, Daley R. Behavior of the myocardium in health and disease as studied by coronary sinus catheterization. *Am J Med* 1951; 10(6):711-718.

(202) Daley R, McMillan I, Gorlin R. Mitral incompetence in experimental auricular fibrillation. *Lancet* 1955; 269(6879):18-20.

(203) Deuchar D. Direct demonstration of a single ventricle. *Guys Hosp Rep* 1952; 101(1):23-31.

(204) Deuchar D, Zak G. Cardiac catheterization in congenital heart disease. I. *Guys Hosp Rep* 1952; 101(1):1-22.

(205) Deuchar D, Venner A. The blood pressure during cardiac massage in man. *Br Med J* 1953; 2(4828):134-135.

(206) Campbell M, Deuchar D. The left-sided superior vena cava. *Br Heart J* 1954; 16(4):423-439.

(207) Talbot S, Deuchar D, Davis F, Scarborough W. The aperiodic ballistocardiograph. *Bull Johns Hopkins Hosp* 1954; 94(1):27-33.

(208) Deuchar D, Talbot S, Scarborough W. Some observations on the relation of the high-frequency bed ballistocardiogram to that obtained from an aperiodic bed. *Circulation* 1955; 11(2):228-239.

(209) Dow J. The venographic localization of incompetent communicating veins in the leg. *Br J Radiol* 1951; 24(280):182-192.

(210) Dow J. Venography of the leg with particular reference to acute deep thrombophlebitis and to gravitational ulceration. *J Fac Radiol* 1951; 2(3):180-205.

(211) Dow J. The venographic diagnosis of the method of recurrence of varicose veins. *Br J Radiol* 1952; 25(295):382-386.

(212) Dubost C, Allary M, Oeconomus N. Resection of an aneurysm of the abdominal aorta: reestablishment of the continuity by a preserved human arterial graft, with result after five months. *AMA Arch Surg* 1952; 64(3):405-408.

(213) Brunsdon D, Enticknap J, Milstein B. A case of subacute bacterial

endocarditis due to Pseudomonas pyocyanea complicating valvotomy for advanced mitral stenosis. *Guys Hosp Rep* 1953; 102(4):303-312.

(214) Enticknap J. Bicuspid pulmonary valve in association with calcific aortic stenosis. *Br Heart J* 1956; 18(4):561-562.

(215) Brotmacher L, Fleming P. The diagnosis by cardiac catheterization of superior mediastinal anomalous pulmonary veins. *Guys Hosp Rep* 1957; 106(4):264-267.

(216) Foxon G. Circulation in the frog. *Nature* 1947; 159(4033):236.

(217) Foxon G, Walls E. The radiographic demonstration of the mode of action of the heart of the frog. *J Anat* 1947; 81(1):111-117.

(218) Foxon G. A simple apparatus for making rapid serial radiographs of small objects. *Br J Radiol* 1948; 21(246):301-304.

(219) Foxon G, Griffith J, Price M. Cineradiographic techniques. *Br J Radiol* 1955; 28(330):336-338.

(220) Kelsey Fry I. Primary decortication in the treatment of acute empyema. *Guy's Hospital Reports* 1948; 97:108-112.

(221) Kelsey Fry I, Earl C. Report on a preliminary investigation into the incidence of inhalation of blood and other debris during dental extractions in the upright position. *Guys Hosp Rep* 1950; 99:41-47.

(222) Gardner F. Angiocardiography. *Postgrad Med J* 1949; 25(289):553-64, illust.

(223) Campbell M, Gardner F, Reynolds G. Cor biloculare. *Br Heart J* 1952; 14(3):317-324.

(224) Gorlin R, Gorlin S. Hydraulic formula for calculation of the area of the stenotic mitral valve, other cardiac valves, and central circulatory shunts. I. *Am Heart J* 1951; 41(1):1-29.

(225) Hills T. Note on an apparatus for angiocardiography. *Br J Radiol* 1948; 21(250):511.

(226) Hills T, Stanford R. The problem of excessive radiation during routine investigations of the heart. *Br Heart J* 1950; 12(1):45-53.

(227) Rink EH, Helliwell PJ, Hutton AM. Anaesthesia for operations for the relief of congenital pulmonary stenosis. *Guy's Hospital Reports* 1948; 97:48-63.

(228) Hills T. Mechanical and physical problems of angiocardiography. *Br J Radiol* 1950; 23(269):279-281.

(229) Hills T, Falconer M. The value of arteriography. *Trans Med Soc Lond* 1953; 69:164-170.

(230) Hoffman P. The history of radiology in the UK since 1895. www bshr org uk/journals/018%20RHHCT%20Journal%2018%202002 pdf [2002 :[9]

(231) Holling H, Zak G. Cardiac catheterization in the diagnosis of congenital heart disease. *Br Heart J* 1950; 12(2):153-182.

(232) Holling H. The pulmonary circulation. *Guys Hosp Gaz* 1951; 65(1644):271-277.

(233) Holling H. Compensatory mechanisms for the anoxia of cyanotic congenital heart disease. *Clin Sci* 1952; 11(3):283-295.

(234) Holling H. Cardiovascular research and the surgery of the heart. *Br Med Bull* 1952; 8(4):358-362.

(235) Holling H, Macdonald I, OHalloran J, Venner A. Reliability of a spectrophotometric method of estimating blood oxygen. *J Appl Physiol* 1955; 8(3):249-254.

(236) Jordaan M. [Surgery of the great vessels of heart]. S Afr Med J 1953; 27(2):37-41.

(237) Jordaan M, Muller H. Surgical correction of aortic stenosis. *S Afr Med J* 1954; 28(42):881-884.

(238) Jordaan M. [Mitral stenosis; experience with my first 100 cases of mitral valvulotomy]. S Afr Med J 1954; 28(19):391-394.

(239) Campbell M, Kauntze R. Congenital aortic valvular stenosis. *Br Heart J* 1953; 15(2):179-194.

(240) Cane C, Kauntze R. Acute aortic valve regurgitation. *Guys Hosp Rep* 1956; 105(2):197-204.

(241) McGregor M. The genesis of the electrocardiogram of right ventricular hypertrophy. *Br Heart J* 1950; 12(4):351-359.

(242) McMillan I, Melrose D, Lynn R. Hypothermia: some observations on blood gas and electrolyte changes during surface cooling. *Ann R Coll Surg Engl* 1955; 16(3):186-194.

(243) McMillan I. Cardiac resuscitation. *Br Med Bull* 1955; 11(3):229-232.

(244) Barber J, Magidson O, Wood P. Atrial septal defect. *Br Heart J* 1950; 12(3):277-292.

(245) Gorlin R, Matthews M, McMillan I, Daley R, Medd W. Physiological and clinical observations in aortic valvular disease. *Bull New Engl Med Cent* 1954; 16(1):13-23.

(246) McArdle B. Myopathy due to a defect in muscle glycogen breakdown. *Clin Sci* 1951; 10(1):13-35.

(247) McArdle B, Verel D. Responses to ischaemic work in the human forearm. *Clin Sci* 1956; 15(2):305-318.

(248) Wood P, McGregor M, Magidson O, Whittaker W. The effort test in angina pectoris. *Br Heart J* 1950; 12(4):363-371.

(249) Starkey G, Milstein B, . Report of a death following selective angio-cardiography. *Guys Hosp Rep* 1953; 102(3):240-245.

(250) Milstein B, Brock R. The operative management of pulmonary valvotomy for pulmonary valve stenosis with normal aortic root. *Guy's Hospital Reports* 1955; 104(1):1-18.

(251) Milstein B. Cardiac arrest and resuscitation. *Ann R Coll Surg Engl* 1956; 19(2):69-87.

(252) OConnell T, Fitzgerald J. Coarctation of the aorta: A new technique. *Ir J Med Sci* 1950;(298):441-449.

(253) OConnell T, Mulcahy R. Emergency mitral valvotomy at full term; report of a case. *Br Med J* 1955; 1(4923):1191-1192.

(254) Campbell M, Reynolds G. The physical and mental development of children with congenital heart disease. *Arch Dis Child* 1949; 24(120):294-302.

(255) Campbell M, Reynolds G. The significance of the direction of the P wave in dextrocardia and isolated laevocardia. *Br Heart J* 1952; 14(4):481-488.

(256) Campbell M, Reynolds G. Electrocardiographic changes during operations for mitral stenosis. *Cardiologia* 1952; 21(4):642-656.

(257) Reynolds G. The atrial electrogram in mitral stenosis. *Br Heart J* 1953; 15(2):250-258.

(258) Campbell M, Reynolds G. Electrocardiographic changes during operations for pulmonary stenosis. *Br Heart J* 1954; 16(1):57-73.

(259) (259) Rink E. Anaesthesia for cardiac surgery. *Ann R Coll Surg Engl* 1950; 7(2):151-158.

(260) Archer E, Blair SN. Physical activity and the prevention of cardio-vascular disease: from evolution to epidemiology. *Prog Cardiovasc Dis* 2011; 53(6):387-396.

(261) Archer E, Blair S. Dr Roy J. Shephard: A pioneer in physical activity and preventative medicine. *Health & Fitness Journal of Canada* 2011; 4(1):27-29.

(262) Schrire V, Vogelpoel L, Phillips W, Nellen M. Experience with mitral

valvotomy at Groote Schuur Hospital, Cape Town. *S Afr Med J* 1955; 29(48):1108-1114.

(263) Campbell M, Suzman S. Transposition of the aorta and pulmonary artery. *Br Heart J* 1950; 12(2):201-202.

(264) Finnegan T, Trounce J. Depression of the heart by quinidine and its treatment. *Br Heart J* 1954; 16(4):341-350.

(265) Hill L, Verel D. Posture and pressure. *Lancet* 1948; 2(6516):120.

(266) Verel D. Postural hypotension: the localization of the lesion. *Br Heart J* 1951; 13(1):61-67.

(267) Verel D. Observations on the effect of posture on the distribution of tissue fluid in the face. *J Physiol* 1955; 130(1):72-78.

(268) Hope A, Verel D. Further observations on the distribution of red cells and plasma in disease; the low body haematocrit: venous haematocrit ratio. *Clin Sci* 1955; 14(3):501-507.

(269) Hicks DA, Hope A, Turnbull A, Verel D. The estimation and prediction of normal blood volume. *Clin Sci* 1956; 15(4):557-565.

(270) Holling H, Verel D. Circulation in the elevated forearm. *Clin Sci* 1957; 16(2):197-213.

(271) Willis R. The borderland of embryology and pathology. Butterworth; 1958.

(272) Waddell W, Sniffen R, Whytehead L. Influence of blood lipid levels on inflammatory response in lung and muscle. *Am J Pathol* 1954; 30(4):757-769.

(273) Waddell W, Sniffen R, Whytehead L. The etiology of chronic interstitial pneumonitis associated with lipid deposition; an experimental study. *J Thorac Surg* 1954; 28(2):134-144.

(274) Woods A. The electrocardiogram in the tetralogy of Fallot. *Br Heart J* 1952; 14(2):193-203.

(275) Zak G, Brun C, Smith H. The mechanism of formation of osmotically concentrated urine during the antidiuretic state. *J Clin Invest* 1954; 33(7):1064-1074.

(276) Zak G. The role of the nitrite concentration in the estimation of antipyrine. *J Lab Clin Med* 1957; 49(4):623-625.

(277) Treasure T. The safe duration of total circulatory arrest with profound hypothermia. [University of London; 1982.

(278) Treasure T, Naftel DC, Conger KA, Garcia JH, Kirklin JW, Blackstone EH. The effect of hypothermic circulatory arrest time on

cerebral function, morphology, and biochemistry. An experimental study. *J Thorac Cardiovasc Surg* 1983; 86(5):761-770.

(279) Treasure T. The safe duration of total circulatory arrest with profound hypothermia. *Ann R Coll Surg Engl* 1984; 66(4):235-240.

(280) Atkins H. Radical mastectomy. *Br J Surg* 1948; 36(141):87-90.

(281) Atkins H. The effect of endocrines on fibro adenosis. *Br Med J* 1949; 1(4608):750-752.

(282) Atkins H. Fibro-adenosis. *Proc R Soc Med* 1950; 43(12):1060-1061.

(283) Atkins H. The painful nodular breast. *Practitioner* 1950; 165(989):482-487.

(284) Atkins H. Fibroadenosis. *Br J Surg* 1950; 38(150):147-163.

(285) Atkins H. Some points in relation to the nodular breast. *Ann R Coll Surg Engl* 1951; 8(2):141-154.

(286) Atkins H. Pain in the breast. *Lancet* 1952; 1(6702):271-274.

(287) Cutler E, Levine S, Beck C. The surgical treatment of mitral stenosis: experimental and clinical studies. *Arch Surg* 1924; 9:691-821.

(288) Swazey JP, Fox RC. The clinical moratorium: a case sudy of mitral valve surgery. In: Freund P, editor. Experimentation with Human Subjects. New York: George Braziller; 1970. 315-357.

(289) Beck C. Resuscitation for cardiac standstill and ventricular fibrillation occurring during operation. *Am J Surg* 1941; 54:273.

(290) Campbell M. Cyanosis and Morbus Coeruleus. *Guy's Hospital Gazette* 1947; 62(1553):43-48.

(291) Crafoord C, Nylin G. Congenital coarctation of the aorta and its surgical treatment. *J Thorac Surg* 1945; 14:347-361.

(292) The Surgery of Congenital Heart Disease. 1948.

(293) Crafoord C, Brock R, Campbell M. RSM Section of Surgery: Surgery of the Heart and Great Vessels. *BMJ* 1951; i:946-947.

(294) Gross R, Hubbard J. Surgical ligation of a patent ductus arteriosus: report of a first successful case. *JAMA* 1939; 112(8):729-731.

(295) Hollman A. Sir Thomas Lewis. Springer; 1996.

(296) Hufnagel C, Harvey W. Surgical correction of aortic insufficiency. *Surgery* 1954; 35:674-675.

(297) Proudfit WL. John Hunter: on heart disease. *Br Heart J* 1986; 56(2):109-114.

(298) Warden H, Cohen M, Read R, Lillehei C. Controlled cross circulation for open intracardiac surgery: physiologic studies and results of

creation and closure of ventricular septal defects. *J Thorac Surg* 1954; 28(3):331-341.

(299) Ribet M. Surgical treatment of carcinoma of oesophagus and Laurence OShaughnessy. *Thorax* 1992; 47(10):842.

(300) Pate J, Sawyer P. Some elastic characteristics of fresh and freeze-dried aortic grafts. *Am J Surg* 1953; 86(6):653-658.

(301) Pate J, Sawyer P. Freeze-dried aortic grafts; a preliminary report of experimental evaluation. *Am J Surg* 1953; 86(1):3-13.

(302) Potts W, Smith S, Gibson S. Anastomosis of the aorta to a pulmonary artery; certain types in congenital heart disease. *J Am Med Assoc* 1946; 132(11):627-631.

(303) Sawyer P, Pate J. Bio-electric phenomena as an etiologic factor in intravascular thrombosis. *Am J Physiol* 1953; 175(1):103-107.

(304) Starr I. Present status of the ballistocardiogram. *Ann Intern Med* 1952; 37(5):839-866.

(305) Wiggers C. Determinants of cardiac performance. *Circulation* 1951; 4(4):485-495.

(306) Hewitt D, Stewart A. Some epidemiological aspects of acute rheumatism. *Br J Soc Med* 1952; 6(3):161-168.

(307) Hoffman P. The history of angiocardiography in the UK since 1985. The Radiology History and Heritage Charitable Trust [2002 Available from: URL:http://www.bshr.org.uk/journals/018%20 RHHCT%20Journal%2018%202002.pdf

(308) Ishiguro K. Never let me go. New York: Faber and Faber; 2006.

(309) Abrams RC. Kazuo Ishiguros Never Let Me Go: a model of completion for the end of life. *Med Humanit* 2016; 42(1):42-45.

(310) Lawrence C. Definite and Material: Coronary Thrombosis and Cardiologists in the 1920s. In: Rosenberg C E, Golden Janet, editors. Framing Disease. New Brunswick: Rutgers University Press; 1992. 50-82.

(311) Wood P. Pulmonary hypertension with special reference to the vaso-constrictive factor. *Br Heart J* 1958; 20(4):557-570.

(312) Gibbon JH. Application of mechanical heart and lung apparatus to cardiac surgery. *Minnesota Medicine* 1954; March(March):171-185.

(313) Kirklin JW, Dushane J, Patrick R, Donald D, Hetzel P, Harshbarger H et al. Intracardiac surgery with the aid of a mechanical

pump-oxygenator system (gibbon type): report of eight cases. *Proc Staff Meet Mayo Clin* 1955; 30(10):201-206.

(314) Kirklin J, Donald D, Harshbarger H, Hetzel P, Patrick T, Swan H et al. Studies in extracorporeal circulation. I. Applicability of Gibbon-type pump-oxygenator to human intracardiac surgery: 40 cases. *Ann Surg* 1956; 144(1):2-8.

(315) MRC. Surgical shock and some allied conditions. *Lancet* 1917; i(4883):502-505.

(316) Bedford D, Sellors TH, Somerville W, Belcher JR, Besterman E. Atrial septal defect and its surgical treatment. *Lancet* 1957; 272(6982):1255-1261.

(317) Mann W. Campbell, John Maurice Hardman. Royal College of Physicians, Lives of the Fellows [2017 Munks Roll, Volume VI Available from: URL:http://munksroll.rcplondon.ac.uk/Biography/Details/737

(318) Baker C, Brock RC, Campbell M. Valvulotomy for mitral stenosis. Report of six successful cases. *BMJ* 1950; i:1283-1293.

(319) Reinhold J, Nadas A. The role of auscultation in the diagnosis of congenital heart disease; a phonocardiographic study of children. *Am Heart J* 1954; 47(3):405-423.

(320) Reinhold J, Rudhe U, Bonham-Carter R. The heart sounds and the arterial pulse in congenital aortic stenosis. *Br Heart J* 1955; 17(3):327-336.

(321) Mungall I. Kenneth Derwent Allanby. Royal College of Physicians Munks Roll: Lives of the Fellows [2017 Volume IX Available from: URL:http://munksroll.rcplondon.ac.uk/Biography/Details/5318

(322) Kayden H, Steele J, Mark L, Brodie B. The use of procaine amide in cardiac arrhythmias. *Circulation* 1951; 4(1):13-22.

(323) Treasure T, Belcher JR. Prognosis of peripheral lung tumours related to size of the primary. *Thorax* 1981; 36(1):5-8.

(324) English P. Emergence of Rheumatic Fever in the Twentieth Century. In: Rosen C, Golden Janet, editors. Framing Disease. New Brunswick: Rutgers University Press; 1992. 20-32.

(325) Truss L. Eats, Shoots & Leaves. London: Profile Books; 2003.

(326) Ross D. A Surgeons' Guide to Cardiac Diagnosis. Berlin, Springer-Verlag, 1962.

(327) Ross B, Brock R, Aynsley-Green A. Observations on central and peripheral temperatures in the understanding and management of shock. Br J Surg 1969;56:877-882.

(328) Wood P. An appreciation of mitral stenosis. I. Clinical features. Br Med J 1954;1:1051-1063.

(329) Wood P. An appreciation of mitral stenosis: II. Investigations and results. Br Med J 1954;1:1113-1124.

(330) Price F. Textbook of the Practice of Medicine.. London: Oxford University Press; 1st Editions 1-8, 1922-1956.

About Tom Treasure

Born in Islington, London in 1947, Tom Treasure started life not far from where the events of this book were taking shape. His parents had met in wartime London, brought together as part of the workforce to do emergency repairs on bomb damaged buildings and infrastructure, father as site carpenter and mother as the quartermaster at the commandeered Ivanhoe Hotel where the crew were billeted. The family left London for Cheltenham where he attended the Catholic primary school and passed the 11-plus for the Grammar School. His education was interrupted by severe asthma and he was hospitalised for six months. Seaside boarding school with the Christian Brothers was deemed the best solution. After that being a medical student at Guys in London was a welcome escape. Many of the doctors who were members of the Club chronicled in his book were his teachers and mentors. His first resident post at Guys was in cardiothoracic surgery which was his lifetime career from qualifying in 1970 to clinical retirement in 2007. He has been active in professional roles including serving as an elected member of council of the Royal College of Surgeons for eight years and President of the European Association for Cardio-Thoracic Surgery. In the 1990s he took a four-month sabbatical at the Wellcome Institute for the History of Medicine. During training he spent a year each in Canterbury, Cambridge, Newcastle upon Tyne and the University of Alabama but most of his adult life has been in London. He was consultant at The Middlesex and University College Hospitals during the 1980s, at St Georges in the 1990s returning to Guys for the remainder of his career.

Lightning Source UK Ltd.
Milton Keynes UK
UKHW012347180920
370150UK00003B/45/J